D1077940

Chronic and terminal illness:
new perspectives on caring and
carers

Chronic and terminal illness:

new perspectives
on caring and carers

Edited by

Sheila Payne

Caroline Ellis-Hill

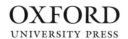

OXFORD

UNIVERSITY PRESS

OXFORD
UNIVERSITY PRESS

Great Clarendon Street, Oxford OX2 6DP

Oxford University Press is a department of the University of Oxford.
It furthers the University's objective of excellence in research, scholarship,
and education by publishing worldwide in

Oxford New York

Athens Auckland Bangkok Bogotá Buenos Aires Cape Town
Dar es Salaam Delhi Florence Hong Kong Istanbul Karachi Kolkata
Kuala Lumpur Madrid Melbourne Mexico City Mumbai Nairobi
Paris São Paulo Shanghai Singapore Taipei Tokyo Toronto Warsaw
and associated companies in Berlin Ibadan

Oxford is a registered trade mark of Oxford University Press
in the UK and in certain other countries

Published in the United States
by Oxford University Press Inc., New York

© Oxford University Press and contributors listed on p. vii

British Library Cataloguing in Publication Data

Data available

Library of Congress Cataloguing-in-Publication Data

ISBN 0–19–263167 5 (Pbk.)

10 9 8 7 6 5 4 3 2 1

Typeset by J&L Composition Ltd, Filey, North Yorkshire
Printed in Great Britain
on acid-free paper by
Biddles Ltd, Guildford & King's Lynn

Contents

List of contributors

Dr Caroline Ellis-Hill
Senior Research Fellow
University of Southampton, UK

Dr Christina Lee
Director of Research
Research Institute for Gender and Health
University of Newcastle
Australia

Professor Mike Nolan
Professor of Gerontological Nursing
University of Sheffield, UK

Professor Sheila Payne
Professor in Palliative Care
University of Sheffield, UK

Dr Karen Rose
Honorary Research Fellow
University of Manchester, UK

Ms Frances Sheldon
Senior Lecturer, Head of Department
Social Work Studies
University of Southampton, UK

Dr Paula Smith
Senior Research Fellow
Institute of Cancer Research
The Royal Marsden Hospital
London, UK

Dr Magi Sque
Director of Studies - MSc Advanced Clinical
Practice
European Institute of Health and Medical
Sciences
University of Surrey, UK

Ms Pauline Turner
Lecturer in Palliative Nursing
School of Nursing and Midwifery
University of Southampton, UK

Dr Bee Wee
Consultant in Palliative Medicine
Countess Mountbatten House
Southampton, UK

Chapter 1

Being a carer

Sheila Payne and Caroline Ellis-Hill

People are social animals. We live, and define, ourselves in terms of our social relationships with others. For example, people are described as mothers, spouses, daughters, sons, grandparents, and cousins. We also define people by their lack of such relationships; for example, as widows, childless, and unmarried. Our social experiences are generally shaped by early interactions within the family and within the wider society (Bowlby 1969). Within these relationships we learn reciprocity, the give and take of normal social life. We learn to be both cared for, and caring, to others. This book is concerned with exploring the nature and determinants of special types of caring relationships, especially those that occur within the context of end of life care, and/or chronic illness. The emphasis will be on those people who are caring for others with acquired physical illnesses or disability, rather than those with mental health problems such as Alzheimer's disease and other types of dementia, as there is little written in this area. We recognize that physical and psychological problems cannot be separated out in a simple way, and for most people the experience of illness and of dying are a complex inter-play between physical, psychological, social, and existential issues.

Before moving on, we feel it is important to define the framework of this book. In this book we have brought together accounts of being a carer for those with chronic and terminal conditions, with research and theorizing from a number of experts within the field. Thus, although the primary focus of the book is in health care, in order to explore concepts around carers and caring fully, we have drawn on academic disciplines and approaches as diverse as health psychology, sociology, social policy, and health services research. The practice-based disciplines of nursing, medicine, rehabilitation, social work, and education have informed the content of this book. Many of the contributors combine the roles of practitioners, educators, and researchers. We do not intend readers of this book to obtain direct advice on how to 'care'. Rather, by exploring the experience and perspectives of those who provide personal, domestic, and/or emotional care to others already known to them by virtue of kinship, co-habitation, or friendship, practitioners and academics can reflect on the nature of caring and its relationship to practice. Therefore, although this book is not primarily concerned with professional caring, we will be theorizing about the interactions between carers and professionals in both health and social services. Another key feature of this book is the focus on caring within a framework of specific life transitions, such as diagnosis of a chronic and potentially life-limiting illness or until death. One of the aims of this book is to consider to what extent caring is special or different when it occurs near the end of life. We will focus on carers providing support to adults rather than children. Some children do, of course, have chronic and terminal illness that require care, and a few children also become carers to adults, usually family members, but these issues are dealt with elsewhere (see Eiser 1990; Segal and Simkins 1993) and are beyond the scope of this book.

In this chapter, we would like to give a brief introduction to the concepts of social support and social relations, drawing predominantly on psychological work, to give a wider theoretical background to the chapters that will follow. As the majority of caring occurs within kinship networks, we will also introduce theoretical perspectives used to explain family dynamics. We will then go on to explore the nature of caring. We will:

1 review why there has been increasing research and policy interest in carers;

2 consider who becomes a carer;

3 consider the work they carry out.

We have deliberately set out by not offering a single definition of a carer. A key tension in our view is the problem of defining what constitutes a carer and what nomenclature should be used. This debate forms a recurring theme in a number of the chapters. We will consider a number of alternative conceptual categories and debate whether 'being a carer' is self-ascribed or merely used by professionals. Finally, we will introduce the context of the book, what we mean by chronic and/or terminal illness, and how current debates within specialist palliative care challenge the previous emphasis on those dying of malignant conditions (National Council for Hospice and Specialist Palliative Care Services 2000).

In short, this book is about 'being a carer'. Specifically it is about how this type of care is investigated and understood by researchers, academics, and practitioners, who may themselves have been carers. The book attempts to offer an understanding of the impact of being a carer of those with chronic and/or terminal illness on the individuals, families, and larger social groups engaged in the process on the one hand, and how individual and social factors shape our expectations on the other.

Social support and social network

In this section we will briefly introduce key theories related to usual everyday relationships, so that readers can put the concepts of caring and carers into a wider theoretical context. This section will only give brief examples from a much wider literature, which readers may want to explore for themselves. We would like to introduce two related but different concepts: social support and social network. Social support has been defined as information leading individuals to believe that they are cared for and loved, esteemed and valued, and belong to a network of communication and mutual obligation (Cobb 1976). A number of different types of social support have been identified. They function in different ways and may involve 'doing for' the supported person, encouraging activity in others, taking responsibility or just 'being there' for others. The following list defines key types of social support.

- Informational support refers to the provision of knowledge relevant to the situation the individual is experiencing.
- Tangible support refers to specific activities that others provide, which are perceived to be helpful.
- Emotional support is the perceived availability of thoughtful, caring individuals who can share thoughts and feelings.
- Affirmatory or validatory support is given when others acknowledge the appropriateness of a person's beliefs and feelings.
- Social affiliation refers to an individual's system of mutual obligations and reciprocal help with other individuals and institutions.

Social support can be differentiated from social network, which is a system of social ties, such as those formed between family, relatives, and friends. Simmons (1994) suggested that there are seven functions of a social network including: intimacy, social integration, nurturing others, reassurance of worth, assistance, guidance, and access to new contacts. Social networks are generally defined in terms of their structural properties including:

- size—the number of people within the network;
- network density—the amount of contact between members;
- accessibility—the ease with which members can be contacted;
- stability over time—the duration of the relationship;
- reciprocity—the amount of give and take in the relationship;
- content—the nature of the involvement in the relationship;
- intensity—the degree of closeness within the relationship.

The mechanism by which social support mediates the effects of stress upon health remains controversial. Two main hypotheses have been postulated: the main effects hypothesis, which suggests that social support is beneficial whether or not the individual is experiencing stress; and the stress buffering hypothesis, which suggests that social support influences an individual appraisal of stressful stimuli. No one psychological model adequately explains all the variance found in the literature. However, it is generally accepted that the extent of the social network is not sufficient to account for the health-enhancing effects, rather it is the perception of the availability of appropriate support and the social skills needed to elicit them, which are the key determinants.

A literature review of social support and breast cancer concluded that social support is important for psychological adjustment and survival for breast cancer patients (Carlsson and Hamrin 1994). Frequently psychological need constitutes the largest number of self-identified needs for both patient and their carer, above physical, financial, informational and household needs (e.g. Hileman and Lackey 1990). The opportunity to confide in others appears to be an important component and a function of social support, although research indicates gender differences in the number of available confidantes, with more women appearing to utilize multiple confidantes (Harrison *et al.* 1995).

Three types of support have been identified for patients receiving radiotherapy: 'being there' (physically, emotional, and spiritually), 'giving help' (instrumental), and 'giving information and advice' (Hinds and Moyer 1997). The authors state that:

> While support was hierarchical in nature, with levels of support linked to the closeness of relationship, it was also multi-faceted.

In other words, different people provided different types of support at different times. Nevertheless, family and friends were found to be the primary source of all types of support. Professional support was mainly perceived to be at an informational level. The authors questioned the appropriateness of professionals providing any support beyond that at an informational level.

Theories of family functioning

The previous section examined social support and social network, and treated 'the family' as one, usually key, source of social support. This makes assumptions that the family functions as the primary source of social support and can be viewed as a stable entity. However, changing demographic patterns, with increasing numbers of divorced and separated people, greater numbers of elderly people, and geographical mobility in the working population, challenge commonly held notions of the family.

The importance of the family to the majority of terminally and chronically ill people can be demonstrated through links between family disturbance and psychological maladjustment, for the family may play a role in exacerbating the stress of cancer as well as easing the burden. Rodrigue *et al.* (1994) found that family disturbance, and perceived quantity and quality of social support, distinguished between good and poor adjustment, for example, and were most likely to predict psychological distress. However, this study was unable to determine any direction of causality in the relationship between family dysfunction and maladjustment, hence the authors conclude that the relationship is probably reciprocal. Different families are likely to respond and cope in different ways when a member has cancer or other type of life-threatening illness, and within a family, members' perceptions may be different.

Researchers have drawn on a number of conceptual categories to investigate and explain family dynamics. The following is a list derived from Payne *et al.* (1999a) in their analysis of family functioning in the context of loss and bereavement. Families vary in the way that they function, for example, the degree to which they are enmeshed. This list does not imply that some families are more functional or supportive than others are, it just recognizes diversity and offers ways of recognizing major differences.

- *Cohesion*—the extent to which family members are enmeshed or connected with each other.
- *Boundaries*—how the family 'system' is divided from the environment.
- *Adaptability*—the balance between pressures to maintain stability and pressures for change.
- *Homeostasis*—maintenance of a steady state.

- *Openness*—the degree to which family members have high levels of exchange with others in their community.
- *Closedness*—the degree to which family members have low levels of exchange with others in their community.
- *Feedback*—the transmission of information about performance, which permits changes and adaptation if necessary.

Kissane *et al.* (1994), for example, defined five types of family interpersonal styles when a member had end-stage cancer along the characteristics of supportive (high cohesion), effective conflict resolution, hostile (high conflict), sullen, and 'ordinary' (moderate levels of expressiveness, cohesion and conflict). Patients' perceptions of family functioning were often different to the perceptions of spouses and offspring. Kissane *et al.* (1994) demonstrated a correlation between family style and psychological health of family members. The two family styles most associated with higher levels of psychological morbidity were those high in conflict and those characterized by a sullen response. From this and similar studies, Kissane and his colleagues went on to develop interventions to support families through the experience of loss and grief (Kissane *et al.* 1998).

Having given a brief introduction to key theoretical approaches that have been applied to social relationships, we would like to move on to focus specifically on caring and to address questions related to the identity of carers such as—why are they becoming important?, who are they?, and what do they do?

Why has there been a growth in interest in carers?

Carers have always been required to care of the sick, the young, and the elderly, and tend the dying. They have also been required to care for the dead, lay-out the body and mourn over it. In the past, and still in many cultures, these tasks are seen to be within the province of the family, friends, and neighbours (Parkes *et al.* 1997). Increasing professionalization has removed some functions almost entirely from the home, such as the undertaker who, in Western countries, usually prepares the deceased body, manages and orchestrates the funeral ritual (Walter 1999). Demographic change in the late-twentieth century, with a marked rise in longevity and increase in the population of elderly people, have highlighted the need for carers of elderly people.

However, carers have not always been a focus for academic research or intervention. Twigg and Atkin (1994) have highlighted the relative invisibility of carers in the social policy agenda of the past. They have proposed two factors that have changed that situation; first, the critique presented by feminist scholarship, which has emphasized the gendered nature of caring; and second, an interest in the role of informal carers in contributing to community based care. Heaton (1999) has argued that there has been a shift in British government policy agenda from care *in* the community to care *by* the community. Referring to the White Paper *Growing older* (Department of Health and Social Security 1981) Heaton writes (1999, p.761):

> In this revised philosophy of community care particular emphasis is placed on the role of family members, as well as friends and neighbours, as the providers of community care; together defined as 'informal and voluntary' sources of support and care.

Heaton (1999) also documented the rise in publications relating to 'informal care' in three bibliographic databases (Medline, Sociological Abstracts, and DHdata) over the last three decades of the twentieth century. She has argued that the discourse of 'informal carer', now usually shortened to 'carer', has emerged since the 1970s. The term 'carer' has become formalized within government policy documents such as the *Carers (Recognition and Services) Act* (Department of Health and Social Services Inspectorate 1996) and has been taken up by voluntary self-help groups such as the Carers National Association. There are marked tensions in current policy rhetoric between the normative assumption that relatives will provide care, and that of 'users' who make informed choices about service up-take and provision. The logical consequence of this being that some relatives may well make conscious decisions not to assume the care-giving role.

Who becomes a carer?

Evidence from the Office of Population Consensus and Surveys (1990) indicates that in Britain there were 6.8 million people defined as carers. The majority were women (3.9 million), with 2.9 million men also providing care. The evidence suggests that women bore the brunt of the burden of care as they provided the majority of personal care, were more likely to be the key (primary) carer, and spent more hours involved in delivering care (Clarke 1995). Carers are predominantly drawn from within kinship networks. The most common being spouses, as they generally cohabit and share the life of the cared for person. Clarke (1995) provides evidence that older spouses spend most time involved in caring activities, and in this group of carers there are few gender differences. Other types of caring relationships are more clearly gendered, with daughters and daughters-in-law, and other female relatives being more likely to participate in providing care (Arber and Ginn 1991). It should also not be forgotten that care-giving is not confined to adults. Segal and Simkins (1993) have documented the impact on children of being involved in providing care for parents with chronic neurological conditions such as multiple sclerosis. While friends and neighbours may be involved in providing additional support, there is less evidence of them becoming involved in the regular provision of care, especially personal care.

There are a number of changing social patterns in Britain and other Western countries that may influence the availability of carers in the future. By the end of the twentieth century, divorce was anticipated to occur in one in three marriages, with remarriage being common (Haskey 1996). Single parenting was also a common feature, with a sizeable minority of all infants being born to unmarried mothers. Serial marriage and step-parenting were therefore common experiences for adults and children (Silva and Smart 1999). This raises questions for the future about how caring will be negotiated in the complex web of relationships resulting from serial marriages and step-parenting. Can it be assumed that ex-partners will feel the same moral responsibility to provide care as existing spouses? Will step-children so readily take on the burden of care for ageing parents? This diffusion of responsibility may be more difficult to manage for health and social care professionals who often seek to identify a single, key carer. However, it may also be a bonus, as this larger network of potentially supportive relationships may compensate for smaller family sizes in each nuclear family.

What do carers do?

The range of roles occupied by carers can vary from covert monitoring of a cared-for person's environment with the aim of anticipating problems and ensuring safety, to 24-h a day hands-on personal care of a highly dependent person. Early research tended to emphasize the physical tasks involved in providing care, using measures that catalogued activities such as the Carer Strain Index (Robinson 1983). The range of personal care tasks involved in providing care for a highly dependent person are likely to include: bathing, toileting, feeding, dressing, and moving the person to ensure comfort and prevent pressure sores. Intimate bodily care and dealing with incontinence are often the most difficult and embarrassing aspects, especially for inter-generational and cross-gender carers. These tasks are often summarized as activities of daily living (ADL). They served to document and represent caring as a 'burden', with the emphasis placed on the negative impact of caring on the carer's physical and psychological health, their limited social opportunities, adverse consequences on their employment prospects, and financial situation. Nolan *et al.* (1995, 1996a) have argued that it is the less visible aspects of caring that are least well recognized and most difficult to accomplish well.

There is plenty of evidence that chronic illness, particularly cancer, affects families as well as the individual with the tumour (e g. Costain Schou and Hewison 1999). Carers have a role in mediating between professionals and patients. For example, they may attend out-patient's appointments to support the patient, obtain information about the disease and treatment, monitor the patient for signs or symptoms of distress. Many carers undertake nursing care tasks, such as giving medication, giving injections, changing wound dressings, cleaning and changing catheters and colostomy bags. While some carers readily acquire these additional skills, some worry about and resent taking on the responsibility, which may subtly alter their relationship with their loved one. Most carers establish good relationships with professionals, but evidence suggests that they may not always understand the roles of different professionals or how to elicit the help they need (Jarrett *et al.* 1999a, 1999b; Payne *et al.* 1999b). For example, a terminally ill person with cancer may be receiving services from a confusing range of providers including the primary care team, the hospital based oncology team, the specialist palliative care team, Macmillan nurses, Marie Curie nurses, social workers, therapists, counsellors, spiritual advisors, home-helps, and volunteers. It is hardly surprising that some patients and carers feel exhausted and overwhelmed by what is often perceived to be a poorly co-ordinated range of services, while for others, especially those with non-malignant disease, such support may not be available.

There are a number of ways to conceptualize and categorize caring. Nolan *et al.* (1995) who built upon the earlier formulations of Bowers (1987), identified eight conceptual categories of caring, including such notions as anticipatory and preventative care. While lists may not be very helpful in a practical sense because types of care may overlap considerably, they are useful in highlighting 'hidden' elements of caring. For example, in caring for a person with a terminal prognosis, the carer may spend time in the early stages, when there are relatively few physical problems, anticipating and planning for deterioration in physical abilities. In a study of patients' and carers' experiences of community based palliative care services in East London (Jarrett *et al.* 1999a), carers indicated the difficulty they had in accessing home adaptations within the time-frame of their partners' advancing cancer, as the following two excerpts illustrate (Jarrett *et al.* 1999a, p.481).

♦ As this patient highlights, the system could be very slow:

> . . . we were waiting for a bath rail. Its sort of takin' a long time to come these things . . . its been a month now . . . need to get into the bath or shower, everything takes so long . . . .

♦ The length of time it can take for patients to receive equipment can sometimes mean that their need has moved on, as this carer illustrates:

> . . . it (stair-lift) won't be much use for him now . . . I doubt he'd make it to the stairs but it will come in handy for me if I'm to stay here . . . .

'Being a carer' represents a social relationship in respect of another person, just as 'being a mother' can only be performed in the presence of an actual or potential child (an expectant mother). Thus the role of carer is performed in relation to another person, even if that person resents or denies the need for care. It is also enacted and attributed to people within encounters with health and social care professionals. Twigg and Atkin (1994) have highlighted the ambiguous position occupied by carers in relation to service provision. They proposed four theoretical models, which typified the response of services to carers.

Carers as resources

Twigg and Atkin (1994) suggest that this model is the taken for granted assumption of most services. From this position, relatives and especially spouses are seen as automatically available to care for the dependent person. Carers are regarded as appendages to the client or patient who is regarded as the 'proper' focus of attention of the professional. There is no onus on professionals to consider the wishes or needs of carers. Within the context of terminal care, it may be taken to imply that the patients' wishes, for example, for a home death, should be prioritized over all other considerations. Nolan *et al.* (1996b) have argued that this way of regarding carers is both morally and ethically indefensible.

Carers as co-workers

An alternative model is to regard the carer as a joint worker with professionals in delivering optimal care for the benefit of the client or patient. While this acknowledges the position of the carer within the enterprise of care, it makes assumptions that there are agreed aims and strategies, for achieving desired outcomes. Thus professional support and services may be directed at enabling carers to continue to provide care, when this might be detrimental to the carer's own health and welfare.

Carers as co-clients

This model explicitly acknowledges that the carer is an individual within his/her own right and has needs, wishes, and roles, which extend beyond the caring role. Recent legislation has recognized that carers have rights to individual assessments. However, it is still potentially pathologizing as it proposes that carers are in need of professional services.

The superseded carer

This category of carer arises in two ways according to Twigg and Atkin (1994). First, as a recognition that for some people, remaining in a caring relationship is potentially dis-empowering. For example, young adults with chronic illnesses, such as cystic fibrosis, who are now increasingly living into their 20s and 30s, may wish to separate themselves from the vigilance and care of their parents (Small and Rhodes, 2001). For these parents, it may be a difficult task to step back from active engagement in their off-spring's life, especially when at the time of diagnosis, the child was probably anticipated to have a limited prognosis. Second, the superseded carer model refers to those people who have decided to relinquish the role of carer. While this is generally thought to apply to carers of elderly people who decide that institutional care is the preferred option, it may also have parallels in palliative care when the burden of caring or acute problems with symptom control mean that admission to in-patient care is accepted (Hinton 1994b).

Carer as expert

In an addition to Twigg and Atkin's (1994) typology of carers, Nolan *et al.* (1995) proposed that carers should be regarded as 'experts' in the care of their dependent person. They have identified that carers build up considerable expertise in the best way to deal with the unique features of their cared-for person, for example, how best to make them comfortable, how to interpret signs of distress and pain in aphasic people. Within this conceptualization, two types of knowledge are legitimized: the individual, lived experience of 'knowing' a person over many years (the carer's knowledge); and the generalized 'professional' knowledge of service providers. Each person has a source of knowledge, which could potentially contribute to the welfare of the dependent person. However, power and knowledge differentials within the professional–carer relationship may mean that there may not be mutual respect for each other's contribution. In particular, carers may be reluctant to challenge a professional's ways of working, especially when the cared-for person is admitted to hospital or other institution such as a nursing home, where professional patterns of working are dominant.

What has been the status of carers in health care?

Linking closely with the previous topic, it appears that there have been changes over time in how health care professionals regard carers. In the past it was regarded as normal for patients to be separated from their relatives and friends on entry into hospital, even children were limited in their contact with parents. Visiting by relatives and friends was restricted both in time and numbers of people (usually two to a bed). The visiting times were organized for the benefit of the institution, rather than allowing easy access for relatives, and were usually strictly control by nursing staff. Hawker (1983), in an ethnographical account of nurses interactions with patients' relatives, identified a range of strategies used by nurses to discourage and limit their contact with questioning relatives, such as the legitimate gait—a purposeful and 'busy' walking style on the ward, with careful avoidance of eye-contact. Relatives were typically regarded as 'in the way' and a nuisance by medical and nursing staff. Latterly relatives, sometimes re-labelled as 'carers', have been regarded as participants in delivering care. For example, it is now common for professionals to invite carers to be involved in discharge planning in elderly care and rehabilitation following stroke (Low *et al.* 1999; Low 2000). There is recognition that carers need skills and knowledge to deliver care. There is also recognition that they should also be willing and informed when making the decision to take up the role of carer. But in reality many relatives take up the care-giver role either by default, as no-one else is available to provide care, or at a time of crisis. It may then be very difficult to relinquish these tasks. Moreover, we would argue that a full partnership model rarely exists, as institutions have structural and financial imperatives that clearly drive the agenda to reduce costs and 'unblock beds' by shifting patients to other sources of care and using the resources of their families.

What has been the status of carers within research in chronic and terminal illness?

A similar pattern in how carers have been regarded and have gained recognition in their own right may also be found in research. To summarize, the responses of carers have been elicited as:

- proxy informants for patients;
- verifying the accounts of patients and/or staff;
- identifying carer's own needs and burdens;
- accounts of the lived experience of caring.

Each of these ways of viewing data derived from carers, makes different assumptions about their status. Each approach tends also to use different types of data-collection methods and analysis. It should be noted that some of the earliest research about the physical and psychological morbidity of people dying in acute hospital wards did not collect the views of their relatives (e.g. Hinton 1963).

Carers as proxy informants for patients

Researchers in palliative care have long faced the difficult problem that their main focus of interest, dying patients, are often too ill, tired, or unwilling to participate in data collection. Moreover, if longitudinal designs are used, a substantial proportion of patients will be deceased before data collection is complete. There have been strong ethical objections to involving dying patients in research (de Raeve 1994). Thus has developed a tradition of sampling the views of bereaved carers to gain an indirect insight into the experiences of patients (Cartwright *et al.* 1973; Cartwright and Seale 1990; Cartwright 1991a; Addington-Hall and McCarthy 1995). Considerable debate has resulted from concerns about the validity of these accounts and the extent to which subsequent psychological process during bereavement may influence the recall of information. Research by Field *et al.* (1995) provides some evidence that these accounts can be regarded as reliable.

Carers as verifying the accounts of patients and/or staff

Within this approach, carer's accounts are collected to verify the responses of the patient and/or staff. For example, Hinton (1979) elicited the views of relatives, patients, and nurses in exploring differences between terminal-care environments (an acute hospital, a nursing home for cancer patients, and a hospice). He sampled 80 married patients who were being treated for malignant conditions and had a terminal prognosis. Assessments of the patient's psychological state, attitudes to their illness, awareness of prognosis, and perceptions of care were compared using rating scales. Correlations between the scores demonstrated that there was most agreement between the views of the spouses, with nurses tending to over-estimate patients' level of distress and under-estimate their level of awareness of their prognosis.

Identifying the needs and burdens of carers

Only relatively recently have researchers recognized the impact of chronic and fatal illness upon the carers, and have considered them as worthy of investigation in their own right. Hinton (1994a) demonstrated the degree of 'burden' and vicarious suffering for relatives as death approaches, such that their levels of psychopathology exceeded those of patients in the last few weeks before death. This approach has tended to use standardized questionnaires or structured interviews to measure constructs such as quality of life, perceived burden, and psychological morbidity. The advantage of this approach is that results become quantifiable and may be compared with other studies. However, there has been a tendency to focus on, and measure, the more negative aspects of caring, with little recognition of the positive aspects. The psychological distress experienced by caregivers within the chronic illness literature has received increasing attention over the last decade. It is often linked to definitions of need. Rosenthal *et al.* (1993) explored the needs of the wives of stroke patients while their husband were hospitalized and found that they wanted to be included in the discharge planning, for example, to know that personnel cared for their husbands and to know the level of activity they were able to achieve. Researchers have also compared psychological morbidity of carers with patient and carer characteristics. Bugge *et al.* (1999) carried out a study to explore the patient, caregiver, and service factors that affected caregiver strain, and found that strain was associated with the amount of time helping a stroke patient, the amount of time spent with the stroke patient, and the caregiver's health. None of the service or patient factors were consistently associated with strain.

Accounts of the lived experience of caring

Qualitative approaches to data collection and analyses have in recent years provided more in-depth accounts of the experience of being a carer. Secrest (2000) has explored the experience of primary supporters following a stroke and suggested that they have a changed relationship with time and their partner, which could lead to a sense of loss and fragility. Habermann (2000) carried out interviews with spouses of people with Parkinson's disease in middle life. Spouses described how the main challenges they were facing were watching their partner struggle and renegotiating their own lives. Contributors to this book have undertaken studies that have employed in-depth interviews to reveal the complex and at times contradictory experiences of caring for a spouse or relative who is chronically ill or dying (see Smith, Ellis-Hill, and Rose, this volume).

What is the context of caring in this book?

At this point in an introductory chapter it is perhaps important to define the context in which caring is delivered. While the words chronic and terminal illness in the title might suggest this is self-evident, a little more thought will uncover a more complex situation.

Chronic illnesses are those for which a cure is currently unavailable. Increasing technological and medical advances over the last two decades are allowing many more people to live with a chronic illness. Also socio-demographic changes in Britain during the last century have resulted in a growing proportion of the population being aged over 65 years, with an especially large increase in those over 85 years. This growing older population is more likely to be living with a chronic illness. The impact of a chronic illness is likely to depend upon a number of interacting variables. They include the nature of the pathology, the resilience and vulnerability of the individual (genetic, physiological and psychological make up), the availability and up-take of health care interventions (e.g. medical treatment, rehabilitation, nursing care), and the social environment. Different conditions are characterized by varying patterns of illness, such as the acute onset of disability following a stroke, the slow but inevitable deterioration of Parkinson's disease, and the remitting and highly unpredictable course of multiple sclerosis. Likewise, within the broad group of diseases called cancers, the impact of illness is likely to be highly variable. Moreover, with many types of cancer, patients and families will live for long periods through a succession of recurrences and treatments, as oncological treatments become more effective at controlling disease. Thus a key feature of most chronic illnesses is living with uncertainty.

Defining terminal illness is also rather difficult as many people live for long periods with 'terminal' conditions. It has been argued that modern medical treatments have, in some circumstances, served to prolong dying. As in chronic illness, the trajectory of dying is uncertain for many conditions, and carers face considerable uncertainty over the length of time they are committing themselves to care and what may be involved in delivering that care. Moreover, the moral imperative to provide the best quality care in a loved one's last illness, may mean that it is very difficult for carers to refuse to provide care initially, to accept respite, and to relinquish care near the end. Family members are aware that for the dying, there are no second chances to get things right.

People with chronic illness are treated by a range of medical specialists, generally depending upon the body system involved (e.g. urologists), or type of pathology (e.g. oncologists), or age (e.g. geriatricians). Palliative medicine as a medical speciality is rather different as it claims expertise in the care of dying people whatever their pathology or age. It may be helpful to explore current debates in palliative care, which seek to offer a definition of this health care area. The World Health Organization (1990) have defined palliative care as 'the active total care of patients whose disease is not responsive to curative treatment', and includes care for the family/carers both before and after death. It includes terminal care but is not synonymous with it. It is generally recognized that palliative care is a central component of all good clinical practice, whatever the stage of illness and wherever the patient is receiving care (Doyle 1997). Primary health care teams are the major providers of palliative care services, as the majority of terminally ill patients live at home for most of the time. Those who provide specialist palliative care have additional expertise and training.

There is limited evidence of the clinical effectiveness of in-patient palliative care, although patients report greater satisfaction with these services compared to standard hospital care (Bosanquet et al. 1997; Addington-Hall et al. 1998; Higginson 1998). Relatively few people die in hospices. Specialist palliative care programmes offer a range of services including in-patient care, home care, day care, outpatient care, and bereavement support, but they are a limited and expensive resource, inequitably distributed and largely limited to those with cancer. There is great national variability in the provision of specialist palliative care services, which have developed in response to local fund-raising initiatives, largely independent of central health-care planning (Clark et al. 1997). Recent changes in specialist palliative care services have resulted in an emphasis on short-term admissions for symptom control and respite care, rather than long-term terminal care (Eve et al. 1997; Higginson 1999). There have been recommendations that specialist palliative care programmes extend their services to those dying from non-malignant conditions (Addington-Hall 1998; National Council for Hospice and Specialist Palliative Care Services 2000). In 2000, less than 5% of their workload was concerned with people with other types of diseases. However, Addington-Hall (1998) has highlighted a number of potential problems including lack of resources, lack of skills, and deskilling other practitioners, if all dying people became within the remit of specialist palliative care.

Evidence from Britain (Higginson et al. 1997) and Australia (Hunt 1997) indicates that there has been a steady rise in deaths occurring in institutions, predominantly hospitals, over the course of the last century. Over half of all deaths occur in acute hospitals, despite concerns that admissions may be inappropriate and quality of care may be poor (Seamark et al. 1995; Higginson et al. 1998). Approximately 32 000 elderly people die in residential and nursing homes in Britain annually (Sidell et al. 1998). Sidell et al. (1998) undertook a three-stage multi-method study involving: a postal survey of 1000 homes in the north-west, West Midlands and south-east of England; interviews with 100 heads of homes; and 12 case studies of the process of care for dying residents. They found variability in quality of care but overall the evidence indicated that standards of terminal care in nursing and residential homes were poor and staff inadequately trained.

In Britain, approximately 26% of deaths occur at home, although the percentage in different parts of the country varies, but over 90% of patients spend the majority of their final year at home (Seale and Cartwright 1994). There is evidence that this is the preferred place for terminal care and death of the majority of people (Townsend et al.

1990; Jones *et al.* 1993), although with increasing longevity, older people may lack family carers and financial resources to enable them to do so. Changing policies and patterns of health and social care have placed greater emphasis on care in the community for patients with end-stage disease (Ingleton 2000). Primary health-care teams are the major providers of palliative care services. General practitioners (GPs) are becoming increasingly skilled at symptom management in the terminal stage of illness (Field 1998). Most of the professional health care received by the terminally ill in the community is provided by district nurses, who often have heavy caseloads and operate under varying levels of support from general practitioners (Goodman *et al.* 1998). Cartwright (1991b) noted that a third of all dying people were visited by a district nurse in 1987, the same proportion as in 1969; however, in 1969 the care provided was over a longer time-span. In contrast, home visits from GPs declined from 88% in 1969 to 77% in 1987. Enabling those patients who wish to, to die at home rather than in hospital, is thought to enhance quality of life, reduce psychological morbidity, and reduce feelings of guilt for carers. This may enable them to cope better with their eventual bereavement (Thorpe 1993; Hinton 1994a; National Council for Hospice and Specialist Palliative Care Services 1998). Primary Care Groups were established in April 1999 but it is not yet clear how they will function to purchase the delivery of palliative care. Home Care Services, provided by Social Services Departments or purchased from the not-for-profit or commercial sectors, play an increasing role in maintaining people who are dying at home and supporting their carers.

However, caring for a dying relative places heavy demand on family members in physical, emotional, and economic terms (Neale 1993). The ability of an informal support network to maintain the individual at home is dependent upon a number of factors such as the material, social, and professional support available to the carer. The most common reason for admission of a terminally ill person to hospital or hospice is a breakdown in the ability of the carer to continue providing the level of help required to allow the individual patient to remain at home (Hinton 1994b). If adequate and appropriate support had been offered to the carer, such admissions may have been avoided.

Introducing the contents of the book

The contributors to this book have written chapters that present not only their recent research, but also a wider theoretical basis to their area of study. We, as editors, are both active researchers, having conducted studies concerned with carers in palliative care (Jarrett *et al.* 1999a; Payne *et al.* 1999b) and stroke (Ellis-Hill 1998; Low *et al.* 1999). We have aimed to present the most recent work in the field. The emphasis of this book is on theoretical and conceptual development within the caring literature. We anticipate that this will be of interest to all students in the fields of health and social care. Although this book is not a practical handbook in 'how to care', all of the contributors have a health or social care professional background and have developed a theory that is firmly based in practice. We have professional backgrounds in nursing (Payne) and occupational therapy (Ellis-Hill) and as editors we recognize the importance of making theory relevant to practice. Therefore each contributor has incorporated a discussion of the practical implications of their work within their chapter. This makes the book of relevance to practitioners, managers, and educators, allowing them to reflect on their practice and challenge common assumptions. Each chapter is introduced by a brief account of its content and ends by offering suggestions and recommendations for practice and professional education. Each chapter can be read as a stand-alone unit of learning, but we hope that the book will be read as a whole.

Chapter 2 builds upon Nolan's previous theoretical work, by proposing that models of caring have failed to adequately conceptualize the positive aspects of being a carer. He argues that previous models of family care have emphasized the distressing and difficult aspects of caring, giving rise to the view that carers are 'burdened', traumatized by the physical and psychological 'load' of care. Instead, he highlights the fact that may family members, particularly spouses, readily taken on the role of carer. While others have argued that this is because they have lacked choice or realistic options, he contends that caring has intrinsic pleasures and rewards. Moreover, by adopting a more positive representation of carers, it could be argued that policy makers and practitioners may view the role in a more pro-active and positive light. Thus carers may no longer be seen as passive and overwhelmed victims of exploitative 'systems' that use their free labour, but as willing and loving care. Nolan supports his claims by drawing upon empirical studies conducted over a number of years with carers of physically frail older people, those with dementia, and learning disabilities. He is careful not to present a romanticized version of caring but demonstrates that carers receive reciprocal support from the cared-for person and the wider community. For example, they feel needed, loved, esteemed, and proud of their contribution. He argues that previous research methods based on checklists of tasks and 'problems', have conspired to hide the more rewarding aspects of care-giving from the attention of researchers. This final point underlines a key theme running through all the chapters, that is the extent to which methodology influences research findings and sets the agenda in what it is possible to 'discover'.

The following three chapters are closely linked. They all use a predominantly qualitative approach to explore aspects of being a carer. In Chapter 3, Ellis-Hill uses narrative analysis to investigate the degree of biographical disruption displayed in accounts of caring provided by spouses of stroke patients. In a longitudinal study, a small sample of patients and carers were followed up over the first year following a first-occurrence stroke. Patients and their spouses were identified in hospital, and three in-depth interviews were conducted over the first year. Ellis-Hill argues that biographical disruption is influenced by the extent to which carer's are able to draw on previous life experiences and expectations. While the majority of the sample of stroke patients made good progress in achieving functional independence, the carers accounts reveal the continuing 'hidden' aspects of caring, namely the way decision-making and assuming 'responsibility' have changed in the family, to fall mainly on the carer. Ellis-Hill argues that current emphasis in stroke rehabilitation upon patient's functional abilities, primarily mobility, is misplaced. Instead she suggests that professionals should listen carefully to the biographical accounts of patients and carers to ensure that rehabilitation goals are compatible with the life-style choices of couples.

Chapters 4 and 5 both focus on carers in palliative care, caring for people dying of cancer. The chapters draw on two longitudinal studies using qualitative approaches, predominantly interviews. One study was conducted in the north-west (Rose) and one in the south (Smith) of England. Both authors are nurses and provide practical suggestions for health professionals arising from their work. Rose documents the labour of caring and goes on to conceptualize it as 'work'. She proposes eight factors that should guide nursing practice: communication, collaboration, commitment, consistency, confidence, consideration, control, and context.

In Chapter 5, Smith addresses the question 'Who is a carer?'. She draws on detailed interviews conducted with people caring for a family member with end-stage cancer at home. Using case-study methodology, she illustrates carer's perceptions of their role and relationships with visiting health professionals. She argues that for some people being a carer is an ascribed label, which they do not readily identify with, while for others it becomes part of their identity. This research illustrates the way interactions between professionals and carers serve to shape expectations and identity. The prioritization of patients' needs are manifest in the difficulty carers have in articulating their own stories and legitimizing their own needs.

Chapter 6 offers an account of carers involved in an acute crisis, from which the outcome is death. Readers may regard this as an odd choice for a book focusing on long-term care. But it is rare for studies of caring in palliative care to include the process of death. There is a sense that caring is completed and no longer required, but this also represents a life transition. This chapter by Sque describes the difficult process for relatives of a previously healthy person who, becoming aware that their family member is dying or has died, have to decide whether to allow organ donation. The transition from normal family relationship, to shocked relative, to bedside carer, to grieving mourner may be accomplished within a few days to a week or more. Sque conducted in-depth narrative interviews with 24 bereaved relatives of organ donors. Using a grounded-theory approach to analysis, she proposes a conceptual model of dissonant loss. She suggests that a series of critical conflicts and resolutions mark the progress of relatives through the acute period of dying and death. The deaths were sudden, complicated, traumatic events occurring in intensive care units. There was considerable ambivalence for relatives in recognizing that their loved one had died despite their warm and florid appearance from artificial ventilation. Sque's work also raises issues about how relatives are engaged in providing care in intensive care units. It raises important concerns about the management of death, the post-mortem care of bereaved relatives and their critical decision-making under stress.

The perspective changes from micro to macro analysis in Chapter 7. Lee reports on a sub-analysis of a major longitudinal survey of 42 000 women representative of the Australian population. Drawing on data from two age cohorts, middle and older aged women, she describes their involvement in caring and the impact this had on their health and welfare. Direct quotes are used to illustrate the wealth of data presented. Lee argues that caring needs to be seen less as a personal issue for individuals who are typically depicted as coping or failing to cope with the tasks involved, and more as a matter of public policy.

Having considered 'being a carer' from a number of different perspectives, using a range of research methods, Chapter 8 offers suggestions for improving the educational experience of health and social care professionals. Sheldon, Turner, and Wee, in an honest and enlightening account, report on their experiences of organizing and delivering undergraduate and postgraduate multidisciplinary workshops, which include the contribution of carers of terminally ill patients. They highlight practical and ethical issues, for example, ensuring that any emotional disclosures by carers are contained and supported, and that new students are also supported in their initial confrontation with the 'messy' and uncomfortable realities of real lives. They argue that careful preparation and clear goals are needs for carers to feel safe and valued.

Finally the book concludes with a chapter in which the themes running through the book are highlighted. We note that there have been three key features in the approaches used by the researchers:

1 a recognition of need to focus on those providing care;

2 a need to understand everyday life rather than purely medical concerns;

3 the temporal changing nature of caring.

We conclude that in order to broaden understanding from a purely burden model of caring, we need to recognize that caring involves making, maintaining, and ending relationships. We move on to discuss relationships between the carer and partner, family and friends, and wider society. We finally conclude with a discussion of the relationship between carers and health and social care professionals, and we introduce aspects that could be considered in order to improve practice.

Summary

There is much that we do not know and do not understand about the needs of carers in chronic and terminal illness. Socio-demographic trends, with increases in the very old, changes in family patterns, increasing female employment, and geographical mobility, all suggest that assumptions can not be made that family carers will be readily available in the future. This will present a challenge in how to deliver good quality home care to those without identifiable family carers. We hope that readers will become engaged by the theoretical debates and empirical evidence presented by the contributors in the following chapters, and not only develop their theoretical understanding but also use this as an opportunity to reflect on practice.

References

Addington-Hall, J. (1998). *Reaching out: specialist palliative care for adults with non-malignant diseases.* National Council for Hospice and Specialist Palliative Care Services and Scottish Partnership Agency for Palliative and Cancer Care, London.

Addington-Hall, J. and McCarthy, M. (1995). Dying from cancer: results of a national population based investigation. *Palliative Medicine,* 9, 295–305.

Addington-Hall, J. M., Altmann, D. and McCarthy, M. (1998). Who gets hospice in-patient care? *Social Science and Medicine,* 46, 1011–1016.

Arber, S. and Ginn, J. (1991). *Gender and later life: a sociological analysis of resources and constraints.* Sage, London.

Bosanquet, N., Killbery, E., Salisbury, C., Franks, P., Kite, S., Lorentzon, M., and Naysmith, A. (1997). *Appropriate and cost effective models of service delivery in palliative care.* Unpublished report, Department of Primary Health Care and General Practice, Imperial School of Medicine at St. Mary's.

Bowbly, J. (1969). *Attachment and loss: Vol. 1 Attachment.* Hogarth Press, London.

Bowers, B. J. (1987) Inter-generational caregiving: adult caregivers and their ageing parents. *Advances in Nursing Science,* 9, (2), 20–31.

Bugge, C., Alexander, H., and Hagen, S. (1999). Stroke patients' informal caregivers. Patient, caregiver and service factors that affect caregiver strain. *Stroke,* 30, 1517–1523

Carlsson, M. and Hamrin, E. (1994). Psychological and psychosocial aspects of breast cancer treatment. *Cancer Nursing,* 17, (5), 418–428.

Cartwright, A. (1991a). Changes in life and care in the year before death 1969–1987. *Journal of Public Health medicine,* 13, 81–87.

Cartwright, A. (1991b). Balance of care for the dying between hospitals and the community: perceptions of general practitioners, hospital consultants, community nurses and relatives. *British Journal of General Practice,* 41, 271–274.

Cartwright, A., Hockey, L., and Anderson, J. L. (1973). *Life before death.* Routledge, London and Kegan Paul.

Cartwright, A. and Seale, C. (1990). *The natural history of a survey: an account of the method-ological issues encountered in a study of life before death.* King Edward's Hospital Fund for London, London.

Clark, D., Malson, H., Small, N., Mallett, K., Neale, B., and Heather, P. (1997). Half full or half empty? The impact of health reform on palliative care services in the UK. In *New themes in palliative care* (ed. D. Clark, J. Hockley, and S. Ahmedhai), pp.60–74. Open University Press, Buckingham.

Clarke, L. (1995). Family care and changing family structure: bad news for the elderly? In *The future of family care for older people* (ed. I. Allen and E. Perkins), pp.19–49. HMSO, London.

Cobb, S. (1976). Social support as a moderator of life stress. *Psychosomatic Medicine,* 38, (5), 300–314.

Costain Schou, K. and Hewison, J. (1999). *Experiencing cancer: quality of life in treatment.* Open University Press, Buckingham.

Department of Health and Social Security (1981). *Growing older.* HMSO, London, Cmnd. 8173

Department of Health and Social Services Inspectorate (1996). *Carers (Recognition and Services) Act 1995: Practice Guidance.* Department of Health/Social Services Inspectorate, London.

de Raeve, L. (1994). Ethical issues in palliative care research. *Palliative Medicine,* 8, (4), 298–305.

Doyle, D. (1997). *Dilemmas and directions: the future of specialist palliative care—a discussion paper.* National Council for Hospice and Specialist Palliative Care Services, London.

Eiser, C. (1990). *Chronic childhood disease.* Cambridge University Press, Cambridge.

Ellis-Hill, C. S. (1998). *New world, new rules: life narratives and changes in self concept in the first year after stroke.* Unpublished PhD thesis. University of Southampton

Eve, A., Smith, A. M., and Tebbit, P. (1997). Hospice and palliative care in the UK 1994–5, including a summary of trends 1990–95. *Palliative Medicine,* 11, (1), 31–43.

Field, D. (1998). Special not different: general practitioner's accounts of their care of dying people. *Social Science and Medicine,* 46, (9), 1111–1120.

Field, D., Douglas, C., Jagger, C., and David, P. (1995). Terminal illness: views of patients and their lay carers. *Palliative Medicine,* 9, 45–54.

Goodman, C., Knight, D., Machen, I., and Hunt, B. (1998). Emphasizing terminal care as district nursing work: a helpful strategy in a purchasing environment? *Journal of Advanced Nursing*, 28, (3), 491–498.

Habermann, B. (2000). Spousal perspective of Parkinson's disease in middle life. *Journal of Advanced Nursing*, 31, (6), 1409–1415

Harrison, J., Maguire, P., and Pitceathly, C. (1995). Confiding in crisis: gender differences in pattern of confiding among cancer patients. *Social Science and Medicine*, 41, (9), 1255–1260.

Haskey, J. (1996). Population review: (6) families and households in Great Britain. *Population Trends*, 85, 7–24.

Hawker, R. (1983). *The interaction between nurses and patients relatives.* Unpublished PhD thesis. University of Exeter.

Heaton, J. (1999). The gaze and visibility of the carer: a Foucauldian analysis of the discourse of informal care. *Sociology of Health and Illness*, 21, (6), 759–777.

Higginson, I. (1998). Palliative and terminal care. In *Health care needs assessment (second series)* (ed. A. Stevens and J. Raftery), pp.183–260. Radcliffe Medical Press Ltd, Abingdon.

Higginson, I. (1999). Evidence based palliative care. *British Medical Journal*, 319, 462–463.

Higginson, I., Astin, P., and Dolan, S. (1997). *Do social factors influence place of death?* Paper presented at the Fifth European Association of Palliative Care Conference, London.

Higginson, I., Astin, P., and Dolan, S. (1998). Where do cancer patients die? Ten-year trends in the place of death of cancer patients in England. *Palliative Medicine*, 12, (5), 353–363.

Hileman, J. W. and Lackey, N. R. (1990). Self-identified needs of patients with cancer at home and their home caregivers: a descriptive study. *Oncology Nursing Forum*, 17, (6), 907–913.

Hinds, C. and Moyer, A. (1997). Support as experienced by patients with cancer during radio-therapy treatments. *Journal of Advanced Nursing*, 26, 371–379.

Hinton, J. M. (1963). The physical and mental distress of the dying. *Quarterly Journal of Medicine*, XXXII, (125), 1–21.

Hinton, J. M. (1979). Comparison of places and policies for terminal care. *The Lancet*, i, 29–32.

Hinton, J. M. (1994a). Can home care maintain an acceptable quality of life for patients with terminal cancer and their relatives? *Palliative Medicine*, 8, 183–196.

Hinton, J. (1994b). Which patients with terminal cancer are admitted from home care? *Palliative Medicine*, 8,197–210.

Hunt, R. (1997). Place of death of cancer patients: choice versus constraint. *Progress in Palliative Care*, 5, (6), 238–242.

Ingleton, C. (2000). Reactions of general practitioners, district nurses and specialist providers to the development of a community palliative care service. *Primary Health Care Research and Development*, 1, 15–27.

Jarrett, N., Payne, S. A., and Wiles, R. A. (1999a). Terminally ill patients' and lay-carers' perceptions and experiences of community-based services. *Journal of Advanced Nursing*, 29, (2), 476–483.

Jarrett, N., Payne, S., Turner, P., and Hillier, R. (1999b). 'Someone to talk to' and 'pain control': what people expect from a specialist palliative care team. *Palliative Medicine*, 13, 139–144.

Jones, R. V. H., Hansford, J., and Fiske, J. (1993). Death from cancer at home: the carers perspective. *British Medical Journal*, 306, 249–251.

Kissane, D. W., Bloch, S., Burns, W. I., Patrick, J. D., Wallace, C. S., and McKenzie, D. P. (1994). Perceptions of family functioning and cancer. *Psycho-oncology*, 3, 259–269.

Kissane, D. W., Bloch, S., McKenzie, M., McDowall, A. C., and Nitzan, R. (1998). Family grief therapy: a preliminary account of a new model to promote healthy family functioning during palliative care and bereavement. *Psycho-oncology*, 7, 14–25.

Low, J. T. S. (2000). *An investigative study on informal stroke carers comparing the impact of two methods of community stroke rehabilitation.* Unpublished PhD thesis. University of Southampton.

Low, J. T. S., Payne, S., and Roderick, P. (1999). The impact of stroke on informal carers: a literature review. *Social Science and Medicine*, 49, 711–725.

National Council for Hospice and Specialist Palliative Care Services (1998). *Promoting partnership: planning and managing community care.* Report from National Association of Health Authorities and Trusts and National Council for Hospice and Specialist Palliative Care Services, London.

National Council for Hospice and Specialist Palliative Care Services (2000). *National plan and strategic framework for palliative care: 2000–2005.* National Council for Hospice and Specialist Palliative Care Services, London.

Neale, B. (1993). Informal care and community care. In *The future of palliative care: issues of policy and practice* (ed. D. Clark), pp.52–67. Open University Press, Buckingham.

Nolan, M., Grant, G., and Keady, J. (1995). Developing a typology of family care: implications for nurses and other service providers. *Journal of Advanced Nursing*, 21, 256–265.

Nolan, M., Grant, G., and Keady, J. (1996a). *Understanding family care: a multidimensional model of caring and coping.* Open University Press, Buckingham.

Nolan, M., Grant, G., and Keady, J. (1996b). The carer's act: realising the potential. *British Journal of Community Health Nursing*, 1, (6), 317–322.

Office of Population Consensus and Surveys (1990). *General Household Survey 1989*, London: HMSO

Parkes, C. M., Laungani, P., and Young, B. (Eds.) (1997). *Death and bereavement across cultures.* Routledge, London.

Payne, S., Horn, S., and Relf, M. (1999a). *Loss and bereavement.* Open University Press, Buckingham.

Payne, S., Smith, P., and Dean, S. (1999b). Identifying the concerns of informal carers in palliative care. *Palliative Medicine*, 13, 37–44.

Robinson, B. C. (1983). Validation of a caregiver strain index. *Journal of Gerontology*, 38, 344–348.

Rodrigue, J. R., Behen, J. M. and Tumlin, T. (1994). Multidimensional determinants of psychological adjustment to cancer. *Psycho-Oncology*, 3, (3), 205–214.

Rosenthal, S., Pituch, M., Greninger, L., and Metress, E. (1993). Perceived needs of wives of stroke patients. *Rehabilitation Nursing*, 18, 148–67.

Seale, C. and Cartwright, A. (1994). *The year before death.* Avebury, Aldershot.

Seamark, D. Thorne, C., Lawrence, C., and Pereira Gray, D. (1995). Appropriate place of death for cancer patients: views of general practitioners and hospital doctors. *British Journal of General Practice*, 45, 359–363.

Secrest, J. (2000). Transformation of the relationship: the experience of primary support persons of stroke survivors. *Rehabilitation Nursing*, 25, (3), 93–99.

Segal, J. and Simkins, J. (1993). *My mum needs me: helping children with ill or disabled parents.* Penguin Books, London.

Sidell, M., Katz, J., and Komarony, C. (1998). *Death and dying in residential and nursing homes for older people: examining the case for palliative care.* Open University, Milton Keynes.

Silva, E. B. and Smart, C. (ed.) (1999). *The new family?* Sage, London.

Simmons, S. (1994). Social networks: their relevance to mental health nursing. *Journal of Advanced Nursing,* **19**, 281–289.

Small, N. and Rhodes, P. (2001). *Too ill to talk? User involvement in palliative care.* Routledge, London.

Thorpe, G. (1993). Enabling more people to remain at home. *British Medical Journal,* **307**, 915–918.

Townsend, J., Frank, A. O., Fermont, D., Dyer, S., Kaman, O., and Walgrave, A. (1990). Terminal cancer care and patients' preferences for place of death: a prospective study. *British Medical Journal,* **301**, 415–417.

Twigg, J. and Atkin, K. (1994). *Carers perceived.* Open University Press, Buckingham.

Walter, T. (1999). *On bereavement.* Open University Press, Buckingham.

World Health Organisation. (1990). *Technical report series 804.* World Health Organisation, Geneva.

Chapter 2

Positive aspects of caring

Mike Nolan

As an unremarkable but nevertheless important principle, the more caregivers are able to define their role as positive, the less caregivers perceive themselves to be victims caught up by inexorable social forces that deny their autonomy. (Opie 1994, p40)

The literature on family (informal) care has grown significantly over the last 30 years, hardly figuring in the 1960s (Brody 1995), yet being one of the most researched topics in social gerontology by the 1990s (Kane and Penrod 1995). Despite such a dramatic change there is a great deal of 'unfinished business' in the field of family care (Brody 1995), with there still being significant gaps in our understanding (Nolan *et al.* 1996). According to Brandon and Jack (1997), the study of family care has suffered from two major preconceptions. First, there is an enduring perception that caring relationships are rarely reciprocal, and are characteriztically unrewarding and almost invariably damaging. As a consequence, the focus of interventions has been almost exclusively on relieving carer burden by applying a therapeutic model in which the professional is seen as the 'expert'. These two factors have had a number of negative effects, casting the recipients of care primarily as burdens, whilst simultaneously promoting and sustaining an 'unshakeable conviction' in the superiority of professional knowledge (Brandon and Jack 1997). Miller and Powell-Lawton (1997) argue that there is an urgent need for a 'corrective balance', in order to rectify existing 'seriously skewed perceptions' and advance both theory and practice in the field of family care (Kramer 1997).

In the context of the present volume, although much of the literature on family care derives from studies of caregivers of older people, and particularly dementia, many of the insights gained are also relevant to chronic and life-threatening illnesses more generally. Not only is the incidence of chronic illness greatest amongst older people but the literature in a range of conditions that typically affect younger age groups, such as multiple sclerosis, spinal injury, and myocardial infarction, also highlights the central role of social support provided by the family (see, for example, Carpenter 1994; Gulick 1994, 1995; Captain 1995; Hainsworth 1995; Lewin 1995; Thompson *et al.* 1995; Sato *et al.* 1996). Moreover, consistent with the wider caregiving literature, it is clear that although the importance of family support in such conditions is widely acknowledged, services to help the family are limited and typically focus largely on the difficulties carers face. Therefore, while there is limited acknowledgement of the need to enrich caring relationships (Captain 1995) and recognition of the importance of focusing on both the hassles and uplifts of care, such approaches are not systematically developed.

This chapter promotes a move away from a 'pathological' model of family care (Twigg and Atkin 1994) by highlighting the range of satisfactions and rewards that most carers experience. The implications of such a shift in emphasis, for the design and delivery of interventions to support family carers, is considered and a case made for the development of a partnership model in which the expertise of both service providers and carers is fully acknowledged. Directions for future research are also suggested, so that the dynamics between carers, those in receipt of care and service agencies can be better understood.

The arguments that are advanced are supported by several years research conducted by the author and colleagues (Nolan and Grant 1992; Nolan *et al.* 1994; Nolan *et al.* 1996; Grant *et al.* 1998; Nolan *et al.* 1998). While this work focused mainly on the needs of carers of physically frail older people, people with dementia, and people with learning disabilities, the results are considered to have wider application in chronic illnesses and life-threatening conditions more generally. However, the relevant emphasis is likely to vary according to important dimensions of the illness experience, such as onset (rapid/gradual), course (constant/progressive/remitting or relapsing), degree of incapacity, and likelihood of death (Rolland 1994). Notwithstanding such variations, many of the central issues are similar and the relevance of the satisfactions of care is also apparent to carers other than those of older people. To set the scene, the chapter begins with a brief consideration of the factors that have brought issues to do with family care into the policy framework and why a burden perspective has predominated.

The emergence of family care

While the exponential growth of interest in family care can be attributed in part to theoretical curiosity among the academic community, one of the major driving forces has been the 'politicization' of caring (Chappell 1996). The widespread adoption of a policy of community care, particularly among developed countries (Davies 1995), and the realization that this is predicated almost exclusively on the efforts of family carers (Walker 1995; Banks 1999), has moved family carers from the margins of social policy to a position where their needs are now a major policy issue (Johnson 1998; Heaton 1999).

This has been reflected in the United Kingdom (UK) by the enactment of legislation (the *Carers Recognition and Services Act* 1995), which, in principle at least, affords family carers the right to an assessment of their needs. However, despite its good intentions, several major recent studies have indicated that the Act has had a limited impact, and has been introduced in an *ad hoc* and piecemeal fashion. Therefore, although assessment is recognized as the key to the development of sensitive and appropriate services (Social Services Inspectorate 1995), assessment practice is poorly developed, and is frequently little more than a 'matter of chance' (Fruin 1998). Carers' needs are often assessed without them even being aware of it and there is little evidence of an explicit and theoretically robust rationale for the assessment process (Fruin 1998). Moreover, despite the current rhetoric, a user perspective still dominates (Heaton *et al.* 1999), with carers' needs not being embedded into the mainstream thinking of many practitioners (Banks 1999). Widespread concern over the limitations of the Carers Act resulted in the launch of the Carers National Strategy (DoH 1999), which is intended to empower family carers and ensure that those who wish to care are enabled to do so without detriment to their health or limitations to their opportunities to participate fully in society.

However, while there now appears to be the political will to improve the lot of family carers, as Chappell (1996) notes, there has to be a more thorough understanding of the nature of caregiving if policy makers and practitioners are to make legitimate assumptions about their needs. This will mean questioning the perceived wisdom about the burdensome nature of caregiving and the consequent goal of interventions of maintaining family carers in their role by relieving the stress they experience.

Moving beyond burden

The high profile of burden within the caregiving literature can best be understood in terms of two sets of concerns. The first was the desire amongst feminists to explore and articulate gender disadvantage in society. The second arose from interest among social gerontologists fuelled by early empirical research that highlighted the difficulties and stresses that carers often face. In a new and emerging field of study, burden provided a rich seam for exploration and it is not difficult to understand its attractiveness to scholars in the field. Indeed it is important to recognize the role that the numerous studies of burden have played in raising the profile of family carers, in both the academic and policy arenas, and to acknowledge the important insights that research into burden has provided in furthering understanding of the situation of carers.

However, as an unintended consequence of the emphasis on burden, a largely pathological view emerged (Nolan *et al.* 1994; Twigg and Atkin 1994) in which caring was characterized as being 'onerous, emotionally demanding, hardly reciprocal and only rarely rewarding' (Ungerson 1987). Despite early empirical support for the belief that caring is invariably negative, being marginal (Gilhooly 1984), such a perception has proved obdurate and has exerted considerable influence on the research and policy agendas.

Notwithstanding the dominance of burden, a counter-view began to emerge in the 1980s that highlighted the potential for caring to provide a source of identity and satisfaction (Davies 1980). As a result of the small but growing empirical evidence base for the existence of caregiving satisfactions, theoretical explanations were also advanced, which began to provide an altogether more sophisticated and rounded picture of the dynamics of family care. Hirschfield (1981, 1983), for example, suggested the concept of mutuality, which she defined as the extent to which carers found gratification and meaning in their situation, and argued that the best caring circumstances were characterized by high levels of mutuality. Conversely, where mutuality was low or absent, then institutionalization of the cared-for person was far more likely. Others have since extended the concept of mutuality, to include any positive quality of the caring relationship based on love and affection, shared pleasurable activities, common values, and reciprocity (Archbold *et al.* 1992).

Stimulated by such insights, studies into the reciprocal nature of caring relationships and the extent to which caring could be seen as 'meaningful' grew in sophistication and volume (Farran *et al.* 1991; Given and Given 1991; Jivanjee 1994; Wenger *et al.* 1996). It soon became apparent that, far from being exclusively burdensome, the vast majority of carers reported some satisfactions, with percentages typically ranging from over 50% (Cohen *et al.* 1994) to well over 90% (Clifford 1990), with most studies indicating that over 80% of carers experience some elements of caregiving as satisfying (Crookston 1989; Summers *et al.* 1989; Braithwaite 1990; Farran *et al.* 1991; Kane and Penrod 1995). Theoretical explanations for the existence of such satisfactions also emerged with reciprocity being a key concept (Nolan *et al.* 1996; Wenger *et al.* 1996), highlighting the subtle and often implicit 'give and take' that defines all family relationships (Finch and Mason 1993), including caregiving (Wenger *et al.* 1996).

In order to explore further the major sources of caregiving satisfaction, Nolan and Grant (1992) devised the Carers Assessment of Satisfactions Index (CASI). This comprises 30 items derived from an extensive postal survey of carers and a number of in-depth interviews. Items were therefore empirically based, being generated from sources of satisfaction identified by carers themselves. In completing the scale, carers were asked to indicate if each item:

- didn't apply to them;
- applied but did not provide a source of satisfaction;
- applied and provided quite a lot of satisfaction;
- applied providing a great deal of satisfaction.

The index can be either interviewer-administered or form part of a postal survey.

In addition to developing the means to explore the empirical bases of caregiving satisfactions, Nolan *et al.* (1996) suggested a conceptual framework for categorizing the satisfactions of care, dependent upon the source of the perceived satisfaction and who benefited. They considered that satisfactions could derive from three main sources:

- the interpersonal dynamic, based on the quality of the relationship between carer and the cared-for person;
- the intrapersonal or intrapsychic orientation of the carer;
- the outcome dynamic in terms of the consequences of caring for the carer and cared-for person.

Similarly, they identified situations in which the main benefit was experienced either by the cared-for person or the carer, and also suggested where benefits were shared. Utilizing this framework they constructed a matrix of caring satisfactions illustrated in Fig. 2.1.

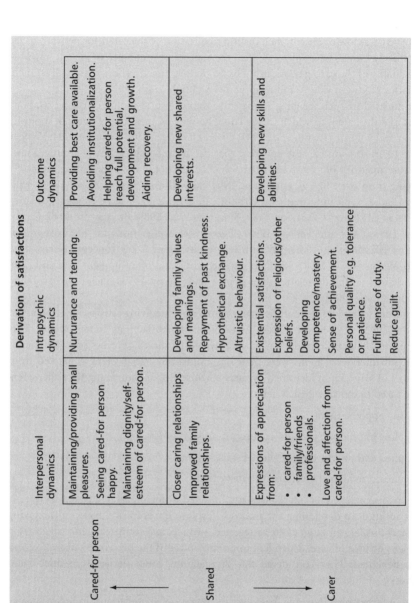

Fig. 2.1 Exploring the satisfactions of care: a completed matrix.

Some quotations from the data reported by Grant and Nolan (1993) help to give life to the often small and seemingly inconsequential acts from which carers experience satisfaction. The quotations below relate to sources of satisfactions arising from the interpersonal dynamic/relationship between the carer and cared-for person.

> When my mother gets pleasure from something I've planned and when I manage to turn her unhappiness to happiness.

> When my husband can remember something about where he has been or what we have done. This means he has enjoyed himself and that makes all the hard work worthwhile.

> Seeing her smile, her pleasure when things go well, my pleasure when she is contented. It's a joy to help her, to always be near her, bringing her a cup of tea in the mornings.

> When my mother puts her arms around me and says she knows what I am doing (although this clarity doesn't last long) and when my aunt says thank you for everything (she always means it).

> When one of her sons or daughters say thank you for looking after their mam, then I feel appreciated and that's all I want.

The following quotations give an indication of satisfactions relating to the promotion of a positive outcome for the cared-for person.

> I find caring very rewarding. I daily see the results of love and loving care. I have a delightful, well-balanced, undemanding and grateful 21-year-old daughter who is admired and loved by all she comes into contact with. My hard work has been very worthwhile.

> Seeing a child who was a limp rag doll finally becoming a human being and knowing that I was a major part of it.

> Bringing my severely handicapped daughter up to be a well-educated, witty, amusing and intelligent human being has been the most satisfying achievement of my life.

Drawing on data collected from 200 carers, mainly, but not exclusively, of people with dementia (see Nolan *et al.* 1996 for a full account), Nolan *et al.* (1996) identified the prevalence of the varying sources of caring satisfactions, as illustrated in Fig. 2.2.

It is important to note that such satisfactions do not relate solely to caring for people with dementia, and recently CASI has been used to explore further the sources of caregiving satisfactions among differing caregiver populations, for instance, carers of people with learning disabilities (Grant *et al.* 1998) and in differing countries, for example, Sweden (Lundh 1999). Although the broad sources of satisfaction were similar, subtle differences were in evidence dependent upon the nature of the disability/illness in question. For example, carers of people with dementia were far less likely to consider as satisfying, working towards small improvements in that person's condition, than were parents of children with learning disabilities. Given the nature of the two conditions, this is a finding that one would predict and adds further to the validity of the conceptualization of satisfactions.

Interestingly, and consistent with the limited other evidence available (Levesque *et al.* 1995), men reported higher satisfaction levels than did women, and spouses were more likely to report satisfactions than were children (Nolan *et al.* 1996). However,

Main beneficiary	Derivation of satisfactions		
	Interpersonal dynamic	Intrapersonal/ intrapsychic dynamic	Outcome dynamics
Cared-for person	Maintain dignity of cared-for person (96) See cared-for person happy (88) Give pleasure to cared-for person (87)	Like to see cared-for person well turned out (91) Cared-for person's needs tended to (79)	Keep cared-for person out of an institution (80) Give best care possible (78) Help cared-for person overcome difficulties (75) See small improvements in cared-for person (48) See cared-for person reach full potential (45)
Shared	Expression of love (89) Closer to cared-for person (49) Closer family ties (39)	Know I've done my best (90) Hypothetical exchange (79) Sort of person who enjoy helping others (78) Repay past kindnesses One way of showing my faith (55)	
Carer	Cared-for person doesn't complain (46) Appreciation from others (56) Appreciation from cared-for person (59)	Provides a purpose in life (25) Stops feeling guilty (31) Grown as a person (43) Test out abilities (45) Provides a challenge (48) Feel wanted and needed (53) Fulfil sense of duty (67)	Widened interests (30) Developed new skills and abilities (42)

Fig. 2.2 Frequency and source of satisfactions experienced by carers.

such differences require further empirical testing, as do the sources of satisfaction to be found in a range of other chronic illnesses such as MS or AIDS. It may also be that there is a need for further theoretical insights into the sources of satisfaction for carers of people who are terminally ill, who are likely to be working within differing time-frames and towards differing goals. Despite this, studies have confirmed the high percentage of carers experiencing satisfactions and have reinforced the importance of satisfactions, both to a more complete understanding of the reciprocal and dynamic nature of family care, and to the development of services to support family carers. It is to this latter area that attention is now turned.

Supporting family carers: incorporating satisfactions

As noted earlier, the main rationale for services to support family carers has been the belief that reducing the burden will relieve stress and therefore enable carers to con-tinue in their role. Such an approach implicitly views carers as resources (Twigg and Atkin 1994) and has also resulted in a simplistic and task-based perception of caring and the genesis of caregiver stress (Grant *et al.* 1998). The general assumption is that those carers who provide the most frequent help are more likely to require support and, as a consequence, assessments of need are usually based on the amount of assis-tance carers provide in terms of activities of daily living (adl). Indeed such is the strength of this belief that entitlement to an assessment under the Carers Act is restricted to those providing 'regular and substantial' care.

Unfortunately there is little empirical evidence to support the relationship between the amount of care given and the degree of stress experienced. Indeed it is increasingly apparent that the nature and quality of relationships between carer and cared-for person are far more significant (Kramer 1997). The pernicious effects of the adl/burden model are such that those most in need of support are frequently not identified (Levesque *et al.* 1995) and, as Brandon and Jack (1997) note, there is an urgent need for a new perspective that recognizes the importance of interpersonal dynamics. It is here that a consideration of the satisfactions of care can help to inform the development of support services for carers, beginning with the identifi-cation of need, through the design of appropriate interventions, to the evaluation of service quality.

In the context of support for family carers it is helpful to think about the influence of satisfactions in three broad areas. These might be termed:

- working for a positive outcome;
- giving good care;
- caring counts.

Working for a positive outcome relates to carers' efforts to maximize the potential of the cared-for person, to improve their quality of life (or death), and to keep the person out of an institution. Giving good care is a related but distinct set of satisfactions underpinned by carers' beliefs that they are in the best position to understand the person's needs and to provide care of the highest quality. Caring counts highlights the importance of recognizing and valuing the contribution of carers and working with them in a genuinely collaborative way. Juxtaposing such a conceptualization of care-giving satisfactions with the temporal sequencing of interventions (identification of need, design and delivery of services, evaluation of quality) has a number of implications for both policy makers and practitioners.

The limitations of existing models for identifying those carers in need of additional support (i.e. the adl/burden model) are increasingly obvious, and a consideration of the satisfactions of care provides an alternative or complementary approach. It is, of course, important to acknowledge that caring is often difficult and that a consideration of the difficulties of care constitutes a core element of the assessment process. However, such difficulties often do not equate directly with the physical aspects of caring but more frequently relate to the behaviour of the cared-for person, such as being constantly demanding, or to carers' own feelings of anger and guilt. Stress is often compounded by a lack of family support and financial resources (Nolan *et al.* 1990, 1996; Schofield *et al.* 1998). Moreover, difficulties and satisfactions are not necessarily opposite sides of the same coin (Kramer 1997) and the presence or absence of satisfactions can be an important factor in identifying those carers in need of additional help and support.

It has been recognized for some time that carers who can find positive aspects to their role are likely to experience better morale and well-being (Gilhooly 1984; Motenko 1989), with Given and Given (1991) arguing that the presence of caregiving satisfactions provides a significant predictor of less stressful situations. In this regard, the balance between 'uplifts and hassles' may provide a better assessment of the caregiving situation than do either alone (Kinney and Stephens 1989). Therefore in situations of high mutuality, carers appear to cope well, even in the presence of objectively adverse circumstances (Hirschfield 1981, 1983; Archbold *et al.* 1992, 1995). Conversely, the absence of mutuality often signals poor caregiving circumstances, even if objectively the situation appears to be unproblematic. Lewis and Meredith (1989) believe that the potentially most fraught caring circumstances are those in which there is no positive feedback, and it seems that those carers who can identify no positive aspects to their role are more likely to be near breaking point (Clifford 1990). On this basis it has been suggested that there is a need to target carers who get no satisfaction (Walker *et al.* 1990; Archbold *et al.* 1992) and either provide additional support or seek alternative caregiving arrangements—low mutuality should be 'taken very seriously' (Archbold *et al.* 1992). Mutuality might be assessed at various points in caregiving but is likely to be particularly important when entry to the caring role is made at a time of crisis, when efforts should be made to gauge the quality of past and present relationships. In circumstances where poor relationships exist, caution must be exercised before assuming that a caregiving relationship should be initiated. In an established caregiving relationship then, the total absence of satisfactions suggests that close attention should be paid to the advisability of continuing the caring relationship.

However, in the present climate of community care, the emphasis is placed almost exclusively on sustaining caring relationships and virtually all interventions are designed with this in mind. While this is entirely appropriate in the majority of cases, more thought needs to be given to which family members should not be expected to care and also as to how, in some circumstances, carers should be helped to relinquish care as an appropriate goal for interventions. This principle is enshrined in the Carers Act and was reinforced in the more recent *Carers national strategy* (DoH 1999), which stressed the importance of not assuming either a family member's ability or willing-ness to care. However, the choice to care or not is rarely part of routine practice, espe-cially at important transition points such as hospital discharge (Henwood 1998; Warner and Wexler 1998), and there is room for improvement in current approaches.

Such considerations may be particularly important in conditions that develop suddenly, for example, or where there is a high likelihood of death. It is often assumed that families naturally wish to care but this is not invariably so, and family members may be reluctant to admit to this in case they are viewed as 'uncaring'. However, Opie (1994) argues that, even in the best of relationships, and in spite of an expressed willingness to care, the full implications of adopting or sustaining a caring role must be fully explored. The use of instruments such as the Mutuality Scale (Archbold *et al.* 1992) or CASI (Nolan and Grant 1992) may prove useful in such circumstances.

Viewed differently, a consideration of satisfactions can also help to inform the design and delivery of more innovative programmes of support for family carers. Consistent with the burden model, the vast majority of interventions to date have either focused on the prevention or reduction of stress. Services such as respite care have therefore predominated and, indeed, respite care or short breaks is the main form of support promoted in the Carers National Strategy. Clearly such services are important, indeed central, but there is also scope for other approaches. A potentially significant, but often neglected, possibility is to actively seek to promote the satisfac-tions of caregiving. This could operate in a number of ways. For instance, Cartwright *et al.* (1994) extolled the benefits of 'enriching' the caregiving relationship by endow-ing it with meaning and pleasure. They suggest that professionals can work with the caring dyad (or family) to either maintain 'customary routines', i.e. activities that provide or have provided sources of pleasure, or conversely to explore 'innovative routine breakers' by identifying new activities that both carer and the cared-for person would enjoy. Such activities need not be expensive or elaborate, indeed they are often seemingly trivial events (Grant and Nolan 1993; Jivanjee 1994). However, identifying them requires an appreciation of previous history and biography. Importantly, it also requires an openness in relationships so that people are able to discuss their feelings and are also encouraged to envision new opportunities. This may be particularly relevant in palliative care situations when the presence of an open-awareness context is likely to facilitate the most productive exploration of possibilities.

As well as enriching relationships, finding meaning in caring can provide an impor-tant coping resource. This has been termed the 'silver lining effect' (Summers *et al.* 1989) with finding meaning in caring being one way of turning a negative situation into a positive one. Therefore working with carers to recognize and identify the positive aspects of their role, possibly using an instrument such as CASI as an aid, is poten-tially both uplifting and empowering. This may be particularly important following the institutionalization of the cared-for person, which often follows a sudden crisis and can engender feelings of considerable guilt amongst carers (Nolan and Dellasega 1999; Nolan 2000). However, such feelings are rarely acknowledged and are even less frequently explicitly addressed. As a consequence, carers may carry a legacy of guilt for several years.

Langer (1993) describes the therapeutic value of assisting carers to 'retell' their story, as this enables them to validate their role. This would seem particularly relevant following placement of the cared-for person in care, when encouraging carers to reflect on their achievements during their years in caring could potentially provide an effective counter-balance to feelings of failure and guilt. This provides an exciting but unexplored avenue for future interventions.

The same logic would apply following the death of a loved one when the facilitation of post-death narratives might do much to highlight all that has been achieved in enabling the person to die in the environment of their choice, in a dignified and peaceful manner.

Another area in which satisfactions can provide important insights relates to the evaluation of the quality and effectiveness of services. Users' experiences of services are to figure more prominently as a quality indicator in the 'new' NHS (DoH 1997) and carers' evaluations of quality are potent indicators of their acceptance of services. Carers often act as the 'arbiters of standards' (Twigg and Atkin 1994) and develop their own sophisticated and sensitive 'measures' (Nolan and Grant 1992). and will either reject or accept reluctantly services that do not preserve the dignity of the cared-for person or are inconsistent with their preferences and wishes (Nolan *et al.* 1996). As Tarraborrelli (1993) suggested, carers find it difficult to accept services from those who know less about the cared-for person than they do. It is therefore crucial that service providers actively engage with family carers and seek to establish their wishes and preferences, together with those of the cared-for person, if services such as respite care are to be accepted more readily (Montgomery 1995).

However, while carers usually consider that they are in the position to provide best care (Nolan *et al.* 1996), this is not invariably the case. In order to provide good care, carers need the requisite knowledge and skills and this may be difficult, especially with the increasingly complex and technical treatment regimes now being given in the home. Carers therefore need to feel confident and competent to give care if their satisfactions are to be optimized. This suggests a reconfiguration of the relationship between professional and family carers, and a reconceptualization of the aims and objectives of interventions designed to support family carers.

The goals and purposes of carer support

If new ways of working with carers are to emerge, a number of considerations need to be brought to bear including the ability to allow carers to exercise genuine choice and to work in partnership with professionals. The nature of the partnership is likely to vary according to the phase of the illness or condition (Rolland 1994). Until recently, policy and practice goals for family carers have rarely been clearly articulated, being underpinned by an implicit model of 'carers as resources' (Twigg and Atkin 1994). Although recent studies suggest that such an assumption still permeates practice (Banks 1999; Heaton 1999), there has been an increasing critique of the 'keep them caring at all costs' approach, with calls for outcomes that move beyond survival and the postponement of institutionalization, to interventions intended to enhance the quality and meaning of life for both the carer and the cared-for person (Lightbody and Gilhooly 1997). Askham (1998), for example, in summarizing the conclusions of a symposium on carer support held at the World Congress of Gerontology in 1997, called for a more catholic approach in which carer support was defined as any intervention that assists carers to:

♦ take up (or decide not to take up) the caring role;

♦ continue in the caring role;

♦ give up the caring role.

This broad definition clearly acknowledges the importance of a longitudinal perspective in which interventions will vary depending on the stage of caring, and is consistent with recent temporal models of caring (see Nolan *et al.* 1996). The ability to exercise a positive choice, and to be empowered to make decisions about whether to take up or relinquish care, is also promoted in the Carers National Strategy (DoH 1999), together with the development of a partnership model in which formal and family carers work collaboratively. The strategy also places particular emphasis on providing support at key transition points, notably at the beginning and end of care, in order to help carers develop the skills and competencies they require. This calls for new methods of working, in which the knowledge and expertise of both professional and family carers is utilized in order to provide the most appropriate package of care.

Brandon and Jack (1997) are highly critical of what they term the 'therapeutic model' of interventions, in which the possession of expertise is vested entirely with professionals, and they argue for more emancipatory approaches. This requires that professionals not only 'think carer' (Wood and Watson 2000) but also value and utilize the knowledge that they hold. However, this is often not the case, as an experienced and expert family carer can be seen as a threat to professional power, with the result that conflict can occur (Allen 2000).

Rather than conflict, what is required is recognition of differing forms of expertise, with Harvath *et al.* (1994) suggesting a balance between what they call 'local' and 'cosmopolitan' knowledge. Local knowledge refers to a carers' unique insight into the experiential world of the patient, with cosmopolitan knowledge representing expertise of a more technical and general nature, usually held by professionals. Nolan (2000) has suggested that carers may possess 'expert' knowledge in a number of areas, such as:

♦ the way the cared-for person responds to treatment;

♦ the way a disease process manifests itself in the cared-for person;

♦ the management strategies that the carer and cared-for person have developed to deal with distressing symptoms or unwanted side-effects of treatment;

♦ the care preferences of the cared-for person;

♦ the routines of the carer and cared-for person;

♦ the particular likes and dislikes of the cared-for person.

All of the above types of 'expertise' are particularly important in chronic illness, as they highlight the variety and heterogeneity, not only of differing conditions but of individual responses to the same disease processes. This is not to deny the relevance of professional knowledge, but a skilful blending of local and cosmopolitan knowledge is essential to ensure optimum care (Harvath *et al.* 1994). Achieving this synthesis requires a different way of working, a fact that is increasingly recognized in a range of disciplines.

For example, the therapy literature has paid growing attention in recent years to the interaction between therapists and family carers, with a number of useful models emerging. Hasselkus (1994), for instance, suggests that in the acute stages of an illness, the professional assumes the lead but that as discharge approaches, the carer becomes far more actively involved, and as they gain sufficient confidence and expertise, the role of the professional should shift to that of facilitator and enabler. Brown *et al.* (1996) also provide a comprehensive framework delineating the potential levels of interaction between family and professional carers as follows:

- no involvement—relationships based on a traditional medical model with a focus on the patient only;
- family as informant—a passive role for the family, purely as a source of information;
- family as therapy—traditional role in rehabilitation where the family assistant is seen as a resource useful in facilitating the rehabilitation process;
- family as co-client—with the family playing a much more active role in goal planning, but not a full member of the multidisciplinary team;
- family as collaborator—included as a full member of the multidisciplinary team;
- family as director—where the family takes the lead role, with the OT acting as a resource and facilitator.

It is models such as these that require further elaboration and testing in a practice context, in order to determine the most appropriate relationship at a given point in time.

One approach that broadly reflects the ethos of empowerment and partnership is the 'carers as experts' model (Nolan *et al.* 1996), which is based on the following principles:

- The primary purpose of the 'carers as experts' approach is to help carers to attain the necessary competencies, skills, and resources to provide care of good quality without detriment to their own health. In this context, helping a carer not to take up or to give up care is a legitimate aim.
- It is essential to consider both a carer's willingness and their ability to care. Some family members may not really want to care but may feel obliged to do so. Conversely, while many family members may be willing to care, they may lack the necessary skills and abilities.
- A comprehensive assessment will include not only the difficulties and demands of caring but also the quality of past and present relationships, the satisfactions or rewards of caring, and the range of coping and other resources, for example, income, housing, and social support that carers can draw upon.

◆ The stresses or difficulties of caring are best understood from a subjective rather than an objective perspective, with the circumstances of care being less important than a carer's perception of them.

'Carers as experts' recognizes the changing demands of care and that skills and expertise develop over time. A temporal dimension is therefore crucial, and this suggests varying degrees of 'partnership'. For carers new to their role, professional carers are likely to be 'senior partners' in possession of important knowledge of a 'cosmopolitan nature', which is needed to help the carer understand the demands they are likely to face. Conversely, experienced carers, many of whom will have learned their skills by trail and error, often have a far better grasp of their situation than professionals, and acknowledgement of this is vital to a partnership approach. At a later stage the balance may shift again so, for example, if it is necessary to choose a nursing home, carers may go back to a 'novice' stage, probably never having had to select a home before. They will therefore need additional help and support. Recognizing and achieving such a balance is the crux of the 'carers as experts' model.

Accepting a 'carers as experts' approach can be difficult for professionals as, in many ways, it challenges their traditional power base, i.e. the possession of unique knowledge (Eraut 1994). On the other hand it can be liberating and open the way for new, and more appropriate, relationships. Schumacher *et al.* (1998) argue that if the aim is to help carers to 'care well', then we need a better understanding of concepts such as mastery, competence, and self-efficacy, and how carers can be helped to acquire them, and also to recognize the power differentials that exist between family and formal carers, and that mediation and negotiation are essential components of mutually supportive relationships (Brechin 1998a, 1998b).

However, despite the extensive existing research in the field of family care and the recent emergence of more holistic approaches that have improved understanding of the reciprocities and satisfactions of carers, gaps in our knowledge remain, with very few studies having explicitly explored the perceptions of both carer and cared-for persons. Moreover, there is clearly a need to better understand the sources of satisfaction in differing chronic illnesses and in a palliative care context if a genuinely holistic view of the dynamics of care is to emerge.

Moving the agenda forward

Certainly one area that would benefit from further conceptual and empirical development is a fuller understanding of the nature and quality of interdependent relationships between those receiving and those providing support, whether family or formal carers. At the start of the 1990s, Kahana and Young (1990) were critical of the existing simplistic models of caring relationships, arguing for the development of a more sophisticated approach that better reflected the dynamic, interactive, and contextual nature of relationships as they evolved over time. Their vision was of an expanded caregiving paradigm that extended beyond dyadic relationships and incorporated the often delicate interactions between cared-for persons, family, and formal caring systems. Unfortunately, the intervening decade has seen disappointingly little work in this area.

However some new insights have emerged that have potential implications for the design and delivery of support. Seale (1996), for instance, suggests that the central dilemma for carers is how to provide support in a way that sustains, rather than undermines, the care-recipient's self-identity and capacity for self-determination. According to Seale (1996), older people strive both to maintain a sense of living a meaningful life and to keep their 'reputation' safe, with reputation being based primarily on being perceived as independent in three important areas: self care; maintaining an orderly physical environment; and sustaining social relationships.

Seale (1996) argues that family carers engage in two sets of activities, one to reinforce perceptions of independence and the other to reduce risk. These are 'surveillance' and 'placement'. Surveillance involves keeping an eye on the older person and 'placement' the initiation of additional support, and ultimately possible admission to alternative care, if safety is unacceptably compromised. However, achieving an appropriate balance between these activities is important, for if older people feel that their self-identity is threatened or their 'reputation' is compromised then they resist offers of support and may consequently be labelled as 'difficult', particularly by formal service providers. According to Seale (1996), carers occupy an ambiguous position, as by providing support they may simultaneously create dependency. The challenge therefore is to provide care in such a way as to maintain a sense of independence and reciprocation in the caring dynamic. This requires creativity and imagination and, particularly for formal service providers, a willingness to conceptualize roles in more innovative ways.

Although Seale's work relates to frail older people, many of whom may have a chronic illness, the arguments are also of relevance to people of all ages with chronic or life-threatening conditions. For example, Rolland (1994) suggests that well-meaning families can wrap ill or dying members in 'cotton wool' and deny them the opportunity to make a full and active contribution. The tensions identified by Seale are equally apparent here and working with all members of the family to maintain reciprocity is clearly important.

Another area in which there is a need for more work relates to gaining the perspectives of both the carer and cared-for person. Cox and Dooley (1996), in one of the few studies to explore simultaneously the views of care-receivers and care-givers, interviewed 91 care-receivers (31 black, 30 Hispanic and 30 white) about their perceptions of their role. They found that most care-receivers found it difficult to accept their need for help due to the high societal value placed upon independence. Consequently, many reported feelings of: being a burden; feeling guilty about needing help; and struggling to maintain independence. However there was also recognition of the need for help and a realization that, if equitable relationships with family carers were to be maintained, then they needed to work collaboratively with those giving care. Care-receivers, therefore, tried:

+ to be as self-caring as possible;

+ not to be too demanding;

+ not to complain too much;

+ to keep their requests to a minimum;

- to let the carer know their help was appreciated;
- to give love to the carer;
- to talk to the carer about their needs.

These data accurately reflect many of the satisfactions reported by caregivers themselves (Nolan *et al.* 1996; Grant *et al.* 1998) and suggest that in many cases care receivers become skilled in maintaining delicate and subtle reciprocities in relationships.

Interestingly, caregivers in the same study (Cox and Dooley 1996) identified a similar set of factors that made caregiving either easier or more difficult. Generally, care-receivers whom it was relatively easy to support:

- tried to help as much as possible;
- provided emotional support to the caregiver;
- were appreciative;
- had a sense of humour;
- were fun to be with;
- did not complain.

Conversely, it was seen as difficult to provide care to someone who:

- resisted the need for help from either family or professionals;
- had no interest;
- was too demanding;
- expected more than the caregiver could provide.

On the basis of their study, Cox and Dooley (1996) identified three general styles of interaction between caregivers and care-receivers:

- positive and pro-active;
- passive and accepting;
- angry, negative and demanding.

They argued that more empirical studies are required to further elaborate upon their results but believe they provide growing support for the need to understand the often delicate and reciprocal dynamics that occur between caregivers and care-receivers. It is important to understand the characteristics and determinants of a positive and pro-active caring style and to promote this as one element of work with chronically ill people and their families

While the above studies signal the need for a more comprehensive understanding of the interactions between family and formal caregivers, recent work from Sweden (Ingvad and Olsson 1999; Olsson and Ingvad 1999) draws attention to the delicate dynamics that often exist between care-receivers and home-carers. These authors describe a diverse and complex range of practical, social, and emotional exchanges that occur. Positive and reciprocal relationships are more likely to develop when home-carers feel appreciated and valued, and have their competencies and skills recognized. Conversely, if care-receivers are seen as: indifferent; negative; nagging; demanding; grumbling or ungrateful, then negative relationships are far more likely.

These authors argue that some 'sharing' of personal experiences is important to the development of positive relationships, and that trust and confidence based on a congruent set of expectations are essential. This is far more likely when there is continuity of relationships over time. Furthermore, as there is often very little in the way of physical improvement among recipients of home-care, Ingvad and Olsson (1999) argue that care-receiver satisfaction with the support they receive is an integral part of job satisfaction for the home-carer, highlighting the need for far greater attention to be given to the emotional climate of the exchange (Olsson and Ingvad 1999).

The congruence between these results, those of Cox and Dooley (1996) and the satisfactions of caring described in a number of studies (Nolan *et al.* 1996; Grant *et al.* 1998), indicate an emerging consensus, but also highlights the need for further empirical work in this area. This is particularly important if formal service providers are to be more fully attuned to the delicate reciprocities in family relations and are also to achieve maximum job satisfaction themselves.

Getting the balance right

While promoting the need to focus more on the positive aspects of caring, Miller and Powell-Lawton (1997) caution that too great an emphasis may provide politicians with a rationale for reducing the support carers receive. However, the advancement of knowledge cannot be impeded by the use to which it might be put and, as this chapter has argued, a greater appreciation of the satisfactions of care has the potential to advance both theory and practice in the area. On the other hand, although there is an increasingly sophisticated appreciation of the dynamics of caring relationships, there is also room for further study. Consistent with caring research in general, most studies into the satisfactions of care have adopted a largely quantitative approach (Kramer 1997) and there is a need to complement such studies with qualitative approaches that 'speak to the caring process or subjective experiences of caregivers' (Brody 1995). This is particularly the case in areas such as stroke or MI where very few qualitative and longitudinal studies exist.

Furthermore greater theoretical insights are likely to emerge if frameworks other than the dominant stress/coping paradigm are employed. An important addition to the satisfactions literature would be the more widespread use of an existential dimension that addresses a broader life perspective concerning values, choices, responsibility, and consequences, in order to appreciate how to transform the caring experience into something meaningful and valued (Farran 1997). A greater focus on the existential aspects of living with chronic and life-threatening illnesses would be consistent with much of the literature in this field. It is such an element that is most often missing from the interactions between professionals and people living with chronic illness, and there is clearly a need for the construction of more elaborate conceptual models.

However, the challenge ahead is more than simply theoretical. The world's population is ageing and with it the incidence of certain chronic illnesses. A global policy aim is to maintain older people in the environment of their choice for as long as possible (International Association of Gerontology 1998) and this is predominantly, but not exclusively, their own home (Victor 1997). Such aspirations cannot be achieved without the support of family carers, yet it is not ethical to sustain family care beyond the point where it is desired or where it results in serious detriment to carer well-being. The chances of many of us being carers ourselves is significant and, if lucky, we will all grow old. If for no other reason than enlightened self-interest, it is therefore to all our advantages that we fully appreciate the nature of family care in order to provide support in the most appropriate and sensitive way. Understanding caregiving satisfactions is key to that process.

References

Allen, D. (2000). Negotiating the role of expert nurses on an adult hospital ward. *Sociology of Health and Illness,* **22**, (2), 149–171.

Archbold, P. G., Stewart, B. J., Greenlick, M. R., and Harvath, T. A. (1992). The clinical assessment of mutuality and preparedness in family caregivers to frail older people. In *Key aspects of elder care: managing falls, incontinence and cognitive impairment* (ed. S. G. Funk, E. M. Tornquist, M. T. Champagne, and A. Copp), pp. 328–339. Springer, New York.

Archbold, P. G., Stewart, B. J., Miller, L. L., Harvath, T. A., Greenlick, M. R., Van Buren, L. *et al.* (1995). The PREP system of nursing interventions: a pilot test with families caring for older members. *Research in Nursing Health,* **18**, 1–16.

Askham, J. (1998). Supporting caregivers of older people: an overview of problems and priorities. In *Australian Journal of Ageing,* **17**, (1), 5–7.

Banks, P. (1999). *Carer support: time for a change of direction.* King's Fund, London.

Braithwaite, V.A. (1990). *Bound to care.* Allen and Unwin, Sydney.

Brandon, D. and Jack, R. (1997). Struggling for services. In *Mental health care for elderly people* (ed. I. J. Norman and S. J. Redfern), pp. 247–258. Churchill Livingstone, Edinburgh.

Brechin, A. (1998a). In *Introduction—research in health and social care* (ed. A. Brechin, J. Walmsley, J. Katz, and S. Peace), pp. 1–12. Sage, London.

Brechin, A. (1998b). In *In care matters: concepts, practice and research in health and social care* (ed. A. Brechin, J. Walmsley, J. Katz, and S. Peace), pp. 170–187 Sage, London,.

Brody, E. M. (1995). Prospects for family caregiving: response to change, continuity and diversity. In *Family caregiving in an ageing society* (ed. R. A. Kane. and J. D. Penrod), pp. 15–28. Sage, Thousand Oaks.

Brown, I., Renwick, R., and Nagler, M. (1996). The centrality of quality of life in health promotion and rehabilitation. In *Quality of life in health promotion and rehabilitation: conceptual approaches, issues and applications* (ed. R. Renwick, I. Brown, and M. Nagler), pp. 3–14. Sage, Thousand Oakes, California.

Captain, C. (1995). The effects of communication skills and raising an interaction and psychological adjustment among couples living with spinal cord injury. *Rehabilitation Nursing Research,* **4**, (4), 111–118.

Carers Recognition and Services Act (1995). Department of Health, London.

Carpenter, C. (1994). The experience of spinal cord injury: the individual's perspective—implications for rehabilitation practice. *Physical Therapy,* **74**, (7), 614–627.

Cartwright, J. C., Archbold, P. G., Stewart, B. J., and Limandri, B. (1994). Enrichment processes in family caregiving to frail elders. *Advances in Nursing Sciences,* **17**, (1), 31–43.

Chappell, N. (1996). The sociological meaning of caregiving and social support: Issues for older people, the family and community. In *Sociology of ageing: interactional perspectives* (ed. V. Minchiello, V. Chappel, H. Kendig, and A. Walker), pp. 148–151. International Sociological Association, Australia.

Clifford, D. (1990). *The social costs and rewards of care.* Avebury, Aldershot.

Cohen, C. A., Pushkar-Gold, D., Shulman, K. I., and Zucchero, C. A. (1994). Positive aspects in caregiving: an overlooked variable in research. *Canadian Journal of Ageing,* **13**, (3), 378–391.

Cox, E. O. and Dooley, A. C. (1996). Care-receivers' perception of their role in the care process. *Journal of Gerontological Social Work,* **26**, (1/2), 133–52.

Crookston, E. M. (1989). *Informal caring: the carer's view.* Cleveland County Council Research and Intelligence Unit, Middlesborough.

Davies, A. J. (1980). Disability, home-care and the care-taking role in family life. *Journal of Advanced Nursing,* **5**, 475–84.

Davies, B. (1995). The reform of community and long term care of elderly persons: an international perspective. In *International perspectives on community care for older people* (ed. T. Scharf and G. C. Wenger), pp. 21–38. Avebury, Aldershot.

Department of Health (1997). *The new NHS, modern dependable.* The Stationery Office, London.

Department of Health (1999*). The carers national strategy.* The Stationery Office, London.

Eraut, M. (1994). *Developing professional knowledge and competence.* The Falmer Press, London.

Farran, C. J., Keane-Hogarely, E., Salloway, S., Kupferer, S., and Wilkin, C. S. (1991). Finding meaning: an alternative paradigm for Alzheimer's Disease family caregivers. *Gerontologist,* **31**, (4), 483–89.

Farran, C. J. (1997). Theoretical perspectives concerning positive aspects of caring for elderly persons with dementia: stress/adaptation and existentialism. *Gerontologist,* **37**, (2), 250–256.

Finch, J. and Mason, J. (1993). *Negotiating family responsibilities.* Routledge, London.

Fruin, D. (1998). *A matter of chance for carers? Inspection of local authority support for carers.* Social Services Inspectorate/Department of Health, Wetherby.

Gilhooly, M. L. M. (1984) The impact of caregiving on caregivers: factors associated with the psychological well-being of people supporting a dementing relative in the community. *British Journal of Medical Psychology,* **57**, 35–44.

Given, B. A. and Given, C. W. (1991). Family caregivers for the elderly. In *Annual Review of Nursing Research,* Vol. 9 (ed. J. Fitzpatrick, R. Tauton, and A. Jacox), pp. 126–141. Springer, New York.

Grant, G. and Nolan, M. R. (1993). Informal carers: sources and concomitants of satisfaction. *Health and Social Care,* **1**, (3), 147–59.

Grant, G., Ramcharan, P., McGrath, M., Nolan, M. R., and Keady, J. (1998). Rewards and gratification among family caregivers: towards a more refined model of caring and coping. *Journal of Intellectual Disability Research,* **42**, (1), 58–71.

Gulick, E. E. (1994). Social support among persons with multiple sclerosis. *Research in Nursing and Health,* **17**, 195–206.

Gulick, E. E. (1995). Coping among spouses or significant others of persons with multiple sclerosis. *Nursing Research,* **44**, 220–225.

Hainsworth, M. A. (1995). Helping spouses with chronic sorrow related to multiple sclerosis. *Journal of Neuroscience Nursing,* **21**, 29–33.

Harvath, T. A., Archbold, P. G., Stewart, B. J., Godow, S., Kirschling, J. M., Miller, L. L. *et al.* (1994). Establishing partnerships with family caregivers: local and cosmopolitan knowledge. *Journal of Gerontological Nursing,* **20**, (2), 29–35.

Hasselkus, B. R. (1994). From hospital to home: family-professional relationships in geriatric rehabilitation. *Gerontology and Geriatrics Education,* **15**, (1), 91–100.

Heaton, J. (1999). The gaze and visibility of the carer: a foucauldian analysis of the discourse of informal care. *Sociology of Health and Illness,* **21**, (6), 759–777.

Heaton, J., Arksey, H., and Sloper, P. (1999). Carers' experience of hospital discharge and continuing care in the community. *Health and Social Care in the Community,* 7, (2), 91–99.

Henwood, M. (1998). *Ignored and invisible? Carers' experience of the NHS.* Report of a UK research survey commissioned by Carers National Association.

Hirschfield, M. J. (1981). Families living and coping with the cognitively impaired. In *Care of the ageing: recent advances in nursing* (ed. L. A. Copp), pp. 159–167. Churchill Livingstone, Edinburgh.

Hirschfield, M. J. (1983). Home care versus institutionalization: family caregiving and senile brain disease. *International Journal of Nursing Studies,* **20**, (1), 23–32.

Ingvad, B. and Olsson, E. (1999). *The care relationship as a dynamic aspect of the quality of the home care services.* Berlin: Paper presented at IVth European Congress of Gerontology.

International Association of Gerontology (1998). Adelaide declaration on ageing. *Australasian Journal on Ageing,* **17**, (1), 3–4.

Jivanjee, P. (1994). *Enhancing the well-being of family caregivers to patients with dementia.* Paper given at International Mental Health Conference, Institute of Human Ageing, Liverpool.

Johnson, J. (1998). The emergence of care as policy. In *Care matters: concepts, practice and research in health and social care* (ed. A. Brechin, J. Walmsley, J. Katz, and S. Peace), pp. 139–153. Sage, London.

Kahana, E. and Young, R. (1990). Clarifying the caregiving paradigm: challenges for the future. In *Ageing and caregiving: theory, research and policy* (ed. D. E. Biegel and A. Blum), pp. 76–97. Sage, California.

Kane, R. A. and Penrod, J. D. (1995). *Family caregiving in an ageing society: policy perspectives.* Sage, Thousand Oaks.

Kinney, J. M. and Stephens, M. A. P. (1989). Hassles and uplifts of giving care to a family member with dementia. *Psychology and Ageing,* 4, 402–8.

Kramer, B. J. (1997). Gain in the caregiving experience: where are we? *Gerontologist,* 37, (2), 218–232.

Langer, S. R. (1993). Ways of managing the experience of caregiving for elderly relatives. *Western Journal of Nursing Research,* 15, (5), 582–94.

Levesque, L., Cossette, J., and Laurin, L. (1995). A multidimensional examination of the psychological and social well-being of caregivers of a demented relative. *Research on Ageing,* 17, (3), 322–60.

Lewin, B. (1995). Psychological factors in cardiac rehabilitation. In *Cardiac rehabilitation* (ed. D. Jones and R. West), pp. 83–108. BMJ Publishing Group, London.

Lewis, J. and Meredith, B. (1989). Contested territory in informal care. In *Growing old in the twentieth century* (ed. M. Jeffreys), pp. 186–200. Routledge, London.

Lightbody, P. and Gilhooly, M. (1997). The continuing quest for predictions of breakdown of family care of elderly people with dementia. In *State of the art in dementia care* (ed. M. Marshall), pp. 211–216. CPA, London.

Lundh, U. (1999). Family carers 2: sources of satisfaction among Swedish carers. *British Journal of Nursing,* **8**, (10), 647–652.

Miller, B. and Powell-Lawton, M. (1997). Symposium—positive aspects of caregiving: finding balance in caregiving research. *Gerontologist,* **37**, (2), 216–217.

Montgomery, R. J. V. (1995). Examining respite care: promises and limitations. In *Family caregiving in an ageing society: policy perspectives* (ed. R. A. Kane and J. D. Penrod), pp. 29–45. Sage, Thousand Oaks.

Motenko, A. K. (1989). The frustrations, gratification's and well-being of dementia caregivers. *Gerontologist,* **29**, (2), 166–172.

Nolan, M. R. (2000). *Getting the most from breaks: the message from research.* Paper given to Crossroads (Wales) Annual Conference, Llandrindod Wells, June 2000.

Nolan, M. R. and Dellasega, C. (1999). It's not the same as being at home: creating caring partnerships following nursing home placement. *Journal of Clinical Nursing,* **8**, 723–730.

Nolan, M. R. and Grant, G. (1992). *Regular respite: an evaluation of a hospital rota bed scheme for elderly people.* Age Concern, London.

Nolan, M. R., Grant, G., and Ellis, N. C. (1990). Stress is in the eye of the beholder: reconceptualising the measurement of carer burden. *Journal of Advanced Nursing,* **15**, 544–55.

Nolan, M. R., Grant, G., Caldock, K., and Keady, J. (1994). *A framework for assessing the needs of family carers: a multi-disciplinary guide.* BASE Publications, Stoke-on-Trent.

Nolan, M. R., Grant, G., and Keady, J. (1996). *Understanding family care: a multidimensional model of caring and coping.* Open University Press, Buckingham.

Nolan, M. R., Grant, G., and Keady, J. (1998). *Assessing the needs of family carers: a guide for practitioners.* Pavillion Publishers, Brighton.

Olsson, E. and Ingvad, B. (1999). The emotional climate of the caring relationship in home care services. Berlin: Paper presented at *IVth European Congress of Gerontology,* 7–11 July 1999.

Opie, A. (1994). The instability of the caring body: gender and caregivers of confused older people. *Qualitative Health Research,* **4**, (1), 31–50.

Rolland, J. S. (1994). *Families, illness and disability: an integrative treatment model.* Basic Books, New York.

Sato, A., Ricks, K., and Watkins, S. (1996). Needs of caregivers of clients with MS. *Journal of Community Health Nursing,* **13**, 31–42.

Schofield, H. and Block, S. Herrman, H., Murphy B., Nankeruis J., and Singh B. *et al.* (1998). *Family caregivers: disability, illness and ageing.* Allen Unwin, Australia.

Schumacher, K. L., Stewart, B. J., Archbold, P. G., Dood, M. J., and Dibble, S. L. (1998). Family caregiving skill: development of the concept. *Image: Journal of Nursing Scholarship,* **30**, (1), 63–70.

Seale, C. (1996). Living alone towards the end of life. *Ageing and Society,* **16**, (1), 75–91.

Social Services Inspectorate (1995). *A way ahead for carers: priorities for managers and practitioners.* Social Services Inspectorate, London.

Summers, J. A., Behr, S. K., and Turnbull, A. P. (1989). Positive adaptation and coping strength of families who have children with disabilities. In *Support for caregiving families: enabling positive adaptation to disability* (ed. G. H. S. Singer and L. K. Irvin), pp. 27–40. Paul H. Brookes, Baltimore.

Taraborrelli, P. (1993). Exemplar A: becoming a carer. In *Researching social life* (ed. N. Gilbert). Sage, London.

Thompson, D. R., Ersser, S. J., and Webster, R. A. (1995). The experiences of patients and their partners 1 month after heart attack. *Journal of Advanced Nursing*, **22**, 707–714.

Twigg, J. and Atkin, K. (1994). *Carers perceived: policy and practice in informal care*. Open University Press, Buckingham.

Ungerson, C. (1987). *Policy is personal: sex, gender and informal care*. Tavistock, London.

Victor, C. R. (1997). *Community care and older people*. Stanley Thorne, Cheltenham.

Walker, A. S., Skin, H. Y., and Bird, N. D. (1990). Perceptions of relationship change and caregiver satisfaction. *Family Relations*, April, **39**, 147–52.

Walker, A. (1995). Integrating the family in the mixed economy of care. In *The future of family care for older people* (ed. I. Allan and E. Perkins). HMSO, London.

Warner, C. and Wexler, S. (1998). *Eight hours a day and taken for granted?* The Princess Royal Trust for Carers, London.

Wenger, G. R., Grant, G., and Nolan, M. R. (1996). Older people as carers as well as recipients of care. In *Sociology of ageing: international perspectives* (ed. V. Minichiello, V. Chappell, M. Kendig, and A. Walker), pp. 189–205. International Sociological Association, Austria.

Wood, J. and Watson, P. (2000). *Working with family carers: a guide to good practice*. Age Concern Books, London.

Chapter 3

Caring and identity: the experience of spouses in stroke and other chronic neurological conditions

Caroline Ellis-Hill

This chapter explores issues of caring and identity in the area of acquired chronic neurological illness. Due to technological advances over the past two decades there are a growing number of people living with chronic illnesses (Gerhardt 1990). It is recognized that following a diagnosis, not only is the person with the illness affected, but the lives of friends and family are also affected (Rolland 1988, 1994). It can be expected that the relative who will be most closely affected is the person's spouse, as s/he shares so much of present day-to-day life, has shared memories, and shared plans for the future. The stories of spouses form the focus of this chapter. The main empirical evidence is drawn from a wider study of the life changes of individuals and their spouses following a stroke (Ellis-Hill 1998). This is supplemented by findings from studies of individuals experiencing other chronic neurological conditions. In this chapter I will discuss important factors relating specifically to chronic neurological illness, which influence the caregiving situation, critique present research on caring in chronic illness, and introduce a new approach/framework based on changes in identity. This approach has been developed to try and understand emotional and psychological challenges facing the spouses of a partner with a chronic acquired disability. The chapter will conclude with practical suggestions relating to this framework.

A key aspect of any chronic illness by its very definition, is its temporal nature. When a person experiences an acute illness, the individual may take up the sick role (Parsons 1951) for the duration of the illness. This proposes that the person relinquishes his/her usual responsibilities and roles in supporting themselves physically, financially, and socially and this is socially condoned as long as they appear to be making efforts to get better (Radley 1994). Once the illness has passed or a cure has been found, life for the individual returns to normal. The effect of the illness is not long-lasting. Chronic illness, by its definition, is incurable; there is no return to the individuals' usual life. The experience of living with a chronic illness has been seen to be analogous to a career (Price 1996). There are many stages and steps through which individuals pass. Morse and Johnson (1991) noted the need to consider the entire duration of the illness and its stages in order to account fully for individual experience. Corbin and Strauss (1988) highlighted differing possible phases of this career: comeback phases, representing the uphill journey to a satisfying workable life with the disability; stable phases, when people and their families are able to maintain a sense of equilibrium and control in life; unstable phases, when new factors arise that need to be taken into account; and downward phases, where people and families have to face deterioration or the approach of death.

The importance of context in understanding the experience of chronic illness has been highlighted by several authors who note the importance of looking at the experience of patients themselves (Conrad 1987; Rolland 1988; Morse and Johnson 1991). This focus highlights the importance of daily relationships between the individual and their family and friends, health and social care professionals, and wider society in general. Morse and Johnson (1991) highlight the need to be responsive to the dynamic changing nature of living with a chronic illness. Differing chronic conditions may share similar features, such as fatigue, unpredictability, and fluctuation in ability. Although all neurological chronic illness cause irreversible life changes, the time-frames and trajectories differ between conditions leading to differing implications for the person and their family; for example, stroke survivors may regain some former abilities, whereas people living with neurological conditions, such as Parkinson's disease or multiple sclerosis, experience gradual decline in their abilities. Time-frames vary greatly; following a diagnosis with Parkinson's disease or multiple sclerosis people can expect to live for many years, whereas the life expectancy following the diagnosis of motor neurone disease is greatly reduced—on average five years. There are two further aspects specific to chronic neurological illnesses that need to be taken into account when considering the caregiving situation. Often the condition is life-threatening; for example, one-third of people die within the first few weeks following a stroke, and the terminal phase of motor neurone disease occurs within only a few years. This has specific implications for spouses who find themselves in a caregiving situation. They are always living with the possibility of death as part of their daily lives. Also, due to damage to the nervous system, a spouse's partner may have a body that is out of control, their partner may loose their memory, have poor concentration, or experience communication difficulties. All of these aspects have a fundamental influence, as they may be seen to have changed as a person. These aspects will affect the relationship between spouse and partner, and also how the partner is viewed by society as a whole.

There is a wide literature on caring in chronic illness (Han and Haley 1999). The majority of studies are carried out from the perspective of a health or social care professional. Vrabec (1997), in a review of caregiver support and burden, found that only 6% of studies took the perspective of the individual within the caregiving situation. When the perspective of the family or spouse are taken into account they are often portrayed in a certain way, for example, Grant and Davis (1997) asked participants to give their own perspective. They asked participants to identify losses following their family members' stroke. By focusing on losses they did not allow positive changes in the self to be described and so reinforced a negative image of caring and disability. Although researchers such as Nolan (Chapter 2, this volume) have highlighted the importance of considering positive aspects of caring, within the literature the caregiving situation is usually described in terms of burden and difficulty.

Current conceptualizations of caring are essentially task-based (Nolan *et al.* 1996). This is reflected in service provision; often when support is provided it is purely practical in nature. However, family and friends have reported that the psychological and social aspects of the caring situation are often those that are more difficult to manage (Anderson 1992; Wellwood *et al.* 1995). It appears that a major reason for inadequacies in service delivery is that the psychosocial aspects of caring situations are still poorly understood. In this chapter I will introduce an alternative way of viewing the caregiving situation. I will explore the situation from the perspective of the spouse and explore how chronic illness impacts on their sense of self and their ideas for their own future. This approach exposes psychological and social aspects, which have not been considered previously.

The impact of chronic illness on biography was first highlighted by Bury in 1982 who coined the phrase 'biographical disruption'. In a study exploring the experiences of people with a diagnosis of rheumatoid arthritis, Bury found that respondents highlighted how their diagnosis separated the person they were in the past from who they were now and who they wanted to be in the future. Charmaz (1983, 1991) highlighted the losses of self that are experienced by people with a chronic illness. Although the concept of biographical change is becoming increasingly used when describing the experiences of people living with a chronic illness, to the author's knowledge this approach has not been applied to the experiences of spouses living with a chronic illness. I have been exploring identity through the use of a narrative approach. It is thought that the creation of personal life narratives create a sense of coherence between our past, present, and future (Hill 1997). An exploration of life narratives forms the basis for the empirical work described later in the chapter. It is felt that the focus on identity is an important way forward because as Radley (1994, p.137) states, 'because sufferers have to live with, manage and explain their problems to others, issues of communication and identity become central to how people cope with chronic illness'. I suggest that this is also important for spouses.

Method

The stories in this chapter are derived from a study of ten couples following a first-time stroke. The ages of spouses ranged from 42 to 81 years and the group consisted of four husbands and six wives from social classes 1–5; one spouse was West Indian, the rest were Caucasian. Their partners had been admitted to hospital following a single stroke; they had been fit and well previously. The ages of the people with a stroke ranged from 46 to 82 years. The least physically affected person had been in hospital for three weeks, experiencing weakness in his arm and leg, and had physically recovered at six months. The most physically affected person had been in hospital for four months, was using a wheelchair at six months and was just beginning to walk at one year. Two of the interviewees were the spouses of partners who had suffered expressive dysphasia—difficulty with verbal expression, although they could write simple messages they had great difficulty in everyday conversation.

Individual life-narrative interviews were carried out with spouses while their partners were in hospital, at six months and one year following discharge. Within each of the interviews, over time the spouses were encouraged to talk about their past life, their present experiences, and their views of the future. The interviews, which were all carried out by the same researcher, were directed as little as possible in order to allow the person to tell their own story. The initial interview covered the following:

- life from childhood onwards;
- the stroke event;
- hospital experience;
- views of the future.

At six months, interviewees were asked about their hospital experience (creating an overlap with the first interview), and their views of the present and future. At one year, areas covered included their experiences from the time of the stroke, moving through the experience of first being at home, and views about the present and future. It was felt that by using an approach that encompassed life in general, undue attention would not be focused on problems and difficulties. The texts were analysed at three levels. First, each interview was analysed to explore themes relating to either the stroke or personal life history at one point in time. Second, the three interviews given by one individual were compared to see how the themes changed or remained the same over one year. Third, the similarities and differences between the stroke themes were compared for all the spouses.

Although the issues highlighted below were all described by spouses, quotes have been included from specific respondents where they seem to capture the flavour of the overall response. They are referenced as follows: line number/time of interview, where 1 = baseline, 2 = six months, 3 = one year, e.g. 1364/1. All names have been changed.

In the following chapter, four key aspects of the life narrative model are highlighted. These are:

1 a sense of fundamental life change;

2 change due to changed relationship with partner;

3 change due to changed relationships with family and friends;

4 impact of professionals.

These four theme are closely interrelated, but have been separated out to ease discussion.

Fundamental life/identity change

When their partners were admitted to hospital, spouses described entering a new foreign world. Their partners had been fit and well previously; they had little experience of hospitals and did not know what to expect. In the early days following admission, although spouses were facing the possible reality of their partners' death, they still had to carry on their lives at home, as well as supporting their partner. Mrs Curtis reflecting at six months said:

There was that dread earlier on, I don't know, a numbness. I just felt void of any feeling really. I can't remember other than that it was just a case of going through the motions from day to day, just to get through each day. (26/2)

Spouses reported how their own sense of self and time became lost. They spoke of sleepless nights, a sense of unreality, putting life on hold, and purely automatic responses to life outside the hospital. They described how they were purely living one day at a time. Wives studied by Rosenthal *et al.* (1993), during their husbands' admission following a stroke, reported similar experiences. All of the 14 wives described a variety of feelings including:

- being as if on a roller coaster,

- having their lives turned upside down;

- feeling emotionally drained when confronting the unknown outcomes of the stroke;

- having difficulty concentrating and experiencing a state of shock.

Stroke by its very nature is sudden and shocking, and spouses were placed in a position where their partners' lives were immediately seen to be in danger. It would be expected that the diagnosis of illnesses such as Parkinson's disease or multiple sclerosis would be a different experience for spouses, as at diagnosis the person does not appear to be unduly ill or disabled. However, Robinson (1988) has highlighted that the diagnosis of multiple sclerosis can have a great effect on potential and present spouses. It is often diagnosed when people are 25–40 years of age and comes at a life-stage when key decisions are often being made; for example, couples have to decide whether to marry, start a family, or whether to let a partner start a new life with somebody else. Robinson also reported how partners may try to do too much in their lives while still physically able, leading to a period of turmoil for present spouses, which some partnerships do not survive. He noted that marital breakdown tended to occur earlier in the disease rather then later when permanent functional problems occur. Habermann (2000) described the life changes of eight spouses in middle life (average age 50 years) following their partners diagnosis of Parkinson's disease. The spouses did not see themselves as changed, they did not see themselves as caregivers as they did not provide any physical care for their partners. The important role for them was to encourage and support their partners in staying active and involved. The ability to see that their partners had a meaningful life, and the opportunity for spouses to carry out their own activities, may have been important factors in these spouses being able to maintain a coherent sense of self. The early stage of the disease may also have had an influence. Carter *et al.* (1998) found that spouses reported significantly more problems as the disease progressed.

For the participants in the stroke study, the sense that time and their identity had changed continued over the period of the study. This longer term fundamental effect was described by Mrs Evans:

It was the feeling of, my life is finished. I just, I just couldn't see beyond, well even now I can't see into any future. I can't see how things are going to turn out. (109/2)

The difficulty in being able to see 'how things will turn out' and the sense of unpredictability have been reported in many studies (Robinson 1988; Charmaz 1991; Duijnstee and Boeije 1998). Battista and Almond (1973) have noted that not being able to plan or move towards personal goals in the future can lead to psychological distress. Spouses in these situations appear to be moving towards the unknown. Mrs Evans highlighted the difficulty of the fundamental change at one year:

> As far as coping [physically] with [husband] really I mean that's been quite straight forward. It's, it's difficult but it's coping with the change in life total change in our lives together 'cause you suddenly come to an abrupt halt you know, everything's just switched off and changed. (1089/3)

The original future that the spouses had anticipated was now changed and they were not sure even after a year what was going to replace it.

Change in relationship with partner

A diagnosis of stroke has been reported by participants to either drive partners apart or bring them together (Secrest 2000). In the present study, spouses' roles and responsibilities as husbands or wives changed, in turn affecting how spouses saw themselves and their opportunities in life. Their usual position and status within the marriage was challenged and their identity as spouses entered a state of flux. There appear to be many factors that contribute to this change in relationship, key changes will be discussed below

Focus in life

The focus in life for each partner within the couple appeared to change following stroke. Anderson (1992), in a survey of 176 stroke respondents and 148 supporters, found that one month after the stroke, the majority of supporters expressed worries about the future and about how they were going to cope; whereas the majority of stroke respondents reported no major worries about the future, seeming to be more concerned with the present. This finding was supported by Ellis-Hill (1998). Following the initial crisis phase, spouses spoke of their worries for the future. The spouses' partners appeared to be living in the present, concentrating on getting their body working again rather than focusing on wider or longer term life issues (Ellis-Hill *et al.* 2000). Nilsson *et al.* (1997) during an in-depth study of 10 people following stroke, reported that stroke respondents became self-centred, suggesting that their personal treatment of the situation required all their mental energy. This has been reported in other conditions. Cox (1992) found, when enquiring about the needs of patients with motor neurone disease, that patients expressed their main need in relation to their physical difficulties; whereas carers expressed a need for support in the areas of the emotional, psychological impact of motor neurone disease, impact of caring, and need for personal psychological support. Therefore it seems that partners have different agendas, which could lead to potential misunderstanding and conflict. The possible influence of the health care system in reinforcing this position will be discussed later in the chapter.

Practical role changes

Within the present study, spouses reported that they not only had to manage their own usual responsibilities but also those usually undertaken by their partner, such as daily household duties, and maintenance of the house, garden, car, and finances. Enterlante and Kern (1995) and Robinson-Smith and Mahoney (1995) found that spouses reported an increase in household work. This was not necessarily a negative experience; in the present study, spouses reported enjoying having the opportunity to learn to drive, managing the finances, or going back to college to study to get qualifications to support their families. Habermann (2000) reported how some of her participants valued their new roles; for example, one spouse developed a career in writing. However, not all of their new roles were positive experiences and spouses also reported worries about the future including organizing family holidays, deciding about house moves, or wondering how their partner would manage if they became ill themselves.

Spouses own activity often became restricted due to the physical support they had to provide for their partners. In the present study, although few spouses needed help with self-care, there were many things spouses had to fetch or carry for their partners, as their partners often found it difficult to move around the house. When people first came home from hospital, relatives took on this 'nursing' role but found it very frustrating when it continued over a long period of time. As Mrs Evans said at six months:

> The minute I sit down and pick up knitting or a book he'll want something um he does try hard not to impose on me too much but he still finds something, can't help himself. (978/2)

This behaviour was occasionally recognized by the stroke respondent themselves. At one year, Mrs Robinson described this difficulty and how the couple managed it:

> G gets up before me because I like him to have his breakfast on his own. So I don't, 'cause as soon as he starts doing something I start—just do this for me, just do so and so, you know what I mean. Whether it's automatic or what it is he's only got to start something and I want something done. So he, he likes to get on and have his breakfast in peace. (278/3)

These practical changes had both a potentially positive impact on spouses' lives and sense of self in that they were exposed to new opportunities and learnt new skills, but also potentially restricting in that their own activity was restricted by the needs of their partner. With stroke, a person's abilities are relatively predictable and stable on a day-to-day basis. Robinson (1988) highlights that this is not the case in multiple sclerosis, where spouse and partner may have differing views about relapses and remissions. Varying judgement about capabilities may cause tensions related to differing expectations. The fluctuations in the ability of a person with Parkinson's disease can also cause difficulties for spouses. Although these practical changes in life have a significant impact on spouses, I suggest that it was the life changes that were hidden that had a fundamental effect on the emotional life of spouses.

Invisible solitary responsibilities

Spouses felt that they had to look out for, and look after, their partners. This not only brought about a fundamental change in the relationship (often wives spoke in terms of returning to a parent–child relationship) but also challenged the spouses' own sense of competency and fairness.

The most onerous responsibility was being responsible for their partners' health—because the original stroke was so unexpected, all signs were often considered to have possible life or death consequences. At six months Mrs Evans described this dilemma:

> But there was a couple of times when he would say to me, my arm feels funny. And that was the exact words he said to me the day he had the stroke. And I'm thinking, oh no. And I'm trying not to show any feelings, and trying to brush it off, and saying, well, what do you mean by funny?, you know, and trying to work out what it was. 23/2

Spouses did not feel that they could share their fears, as they did not want to upset their partners. Spouses had to become 'paramedics' but at the same time did not feel equipped to deal with possible problems. At one year, Mr Robinson described an incident when his wife lost her speech. He called an ambulance, and by the time they had arrived her speech had returned. But as he said:

> I don't know what it was you don't know about medicine well you don't know do you I wouldn't know right from wrong you know. (78/3)

This left the spouses feeling unsure and lacking in confidence in an area that was of vital importance to them. The challenge to their sense of competence increased their sense of vulnerability (Secrest 2000). Cox (1992) reported that many carers have little knowledge available to them about motor neurone disease. Often carers are not prepared for the new roles they have to take on and have to learn by trial and error (Stewart *et al.* 1993).

Spouses practised vigilance in other areas of life. At six months, Mrs Gunner described how she saw her husband as being more vulnerable:

> I do find sometimes I get a bit nervous here I think if anything happened, you know, I wouldn't be able to get B out of the house quick, that type of thing makes you very aware. You look, you check things double to make sure everything's switched off, you know, you see danger. (813/2)

At one year Mr Robinson described how he still had to 'look out' for his wife. He said:

> I mean I've seen her do things I think Christ don't you do that again. I can foresee problems now. I'm always looking to see if there's a problem ahead that she might run into. (1320/3)

Davis and Grant (1994) described how their respondents monitored and evaluated their relatives' condition over time, for example, watching to see how they were managing on the stairs or how they were coping with being with other people. Secrest (2000) found that her respondents reported that their relatives could not be trusted to monitor themselves and needed supervision.

Spouses also took on responsibility for how their partner spent their time. Outpatient rehabilitation was often seen as a time when this responsibility was shared. Mrs Curtis' husband had good physical recovery but severe speech problems. At six months she said:

> He has such an empty life and he does get bored but I don't know what to do to make his life fuller 'cause he's got to do it for himself to a certain extent. You can't do everything for him and I'm really worried about when he stops going into hospital. (343/2)

Outpatient rehabilitation was seen as a way of structuring her husband's week, having some activity that was his own, for which she was not responsible. Habermann (2000) noted that the spouses of partners with Parkinson's disease felt they could cope with the future as long as partners could continue to do things that were satisfying and meaningful to them. Kellet and Mannion (1999) noted that the ability to continue a meaningful family life has a powerful effect on the experience of stress. The sense of vigilance and concern was all-encompassing and formed a constant background to the spouses' lives.

While spouses had to adjust to practical difficulties, take on new vigilance, and occupational roles, they also had to manage their own emotional reactions, which they could not share with others. As mentioned previously, they often hid their fears so as not to upset their partner. In hospital, spouses became the protectors of their partners, as well as putting their partners' needs first. Spouses reported the emotional strain in trying to maintain an 'ordinary' life outside the hospital, when they found themselves in an extra-ordinary situation, with an uncertain present and an unknown future. Mrs Gunner looking back at six months said:

> While I was in hospital I coped and I could do anything for Bob and I would do anything to help him. As soon as I was away from the hospital I went to pieces... it was when I was away from him that I couldn't cope you know, you find your fears when you're away. (436/2)

Spouses often put on a brave face for their partners to create a sense of reassurance.

As part of rehabilitation, spouses had to let their partners struggle to do things for themselves. At the same time, spouses described how they had to manage their own feelings of hurt and loss. As Mr Robinson said at one year:

> ...and I feel sorry for her really, I do really feel sorry for her and all and it upsets me sometimes to see her incapable as she is to what she used to be. (1506/3)

Anderson (1988) described how family members found it was distressing to see their relatives dependent and restricted. Parker (1993) highlighted the intensity of feeling when the cared-for was a spouse. She suggested that when spouses act in a caring role, they are not only caring *for* their partner but also caring *about* them in an intimate way, the nature of the relationship making it difficult, if not impossible, to distance themselves from the experience. Spouses of partners with early Parkinson's disease reported that the most challenging aspects of their lives was to see their partners struggling and becoming frustrated because of the disease (Habermann 2000).

Spouses saw their partners as vulnerable and wanted to protect them; often they did not share their fears with them. Also the emotional hidden work, which they carried out, was not always obvious to the spouses themselves. Spouses found that they had little time for themselves and often could not understand why they were so stressed because they did not seem to be 'doing' very much. As Mrs Evans said at one year:

> Nothing gets done out there [garden] any more. It's silly, because I'm inactive and yet I've got no time. It's a contradiction you know, I'm aware of it and I just can't understand it. I

seem to be at everybody's beck and call but I don't achieve anything and I don't feel as if I'm doing anything. It feels as if anything's just gone by the board. (292/3)

Keeping their worries and fears to themselves must have been emotionally exhausting for the spouses over the long term. Although aspects relating to relationship change have been reported in other chronic conditions, Goldstein and Leigh (1999) note that this is an area that has been neglected in understanding the experience of motor neurone disease.

Changed relationship with family and friends

Spouses reported that relationships with family and friends changed, further challenging their own sense of self. In hospital they appeared to be facing this new situation alone—only very close family members, for example, daughters appeared to be able to appreciate how they were feeling. Denman (1998), in a study of the needs of aphasic partners' spouses, found that although family and friends were often supportive while their partner was in hospital, few were involved later in the day-to-day support of partners. Although maintaining close contact with former friends at six months, Mrs Gunner described how she did not feel able to talk to them as she had previously, as they did not seem to appreciate her experience. She compared the experience of two of her friends whose husbands had heart attacks, which although requiring operations allowed them to get back to work:

Bob had one stroke and they can't do anything to put him right. And yet when you say heart attack people automatically think—waah, terrible. And it is terrible. But they can mend that. And yet they can't mend a stroke. And yet people dismiss strokes, as though it's er not so serious. That's what amazes me. That, that's the thing that really, and, and I find myself, because I think where people don't understand it, they're inclined to think that, what's all this fuss about, why are you still backwards and forwards to the hospital. And you think, well you just don't understand. (429/2)

Kuyper and Wester (1998) found that spouses often expressed disappointment and/or bitterness about the reactions of friends and colleagues to their partners' chronic disease. Spouses appeared to become more isolated from their partner due to a need to protect them, but at the same time did not feel that they could receive emotional support from family and friends.

Also, due to the focus on the medical aspects of life and changes in priority, spouses in the present study reported that their social opportunities were reduced. Mrs Evans reported:

I just felt as though my whole life had slowed right down, and I just felt totally out of gear. I don't know how else to describe it really. He just didn't want to do anything, to go anywhere or, if we did, it was, like usually it was hospital appointments. That would be the only thing we would go out for. But, since that little break we had, I, he's been more positive about wanting to go out. (955/2)

Even when spouses did get out socially they often found that their usual roles were changed—they still felt the need to protect and look out for their partner. Also they occasionally felt the need to compensate for their partner within the new social relationships formed. For example, one spouse spoke of how previously her husband was the life and soul of the party, but that now he was quieter, she had to work harder to keep conversations going. Habermann (2000) reported that the spouses of partners with Parkinson's disease found that often social circles changed over time and often there was an increase in the informal gatherings with close friends—giving more flexibility for their partner when feeling tired or uncomfortable. Due to the change in expectations when out socially, and their own tiredness and potential loss of confidence, often spouses reported a reduction in their own social life as it often did not seem worth all the effort.

As well as family and friends, spouses' situations were often made more difficult due to the invisibility of their life changes and the invisibility of their partners' difficulties with wider society in general. This was highlighted by Mrs Gunner at one year.

> It's a 24 hour a day job really you know. I don't think people realise, they don't. They look at somebody, unless they're sat there all twisted up and his face all distorted like it was in the beginning, then they could see that there was something. Looking at Bob now when he's sat in his wheelchair you think, 'What the hell's he doing in the wheelchair?'. (121/3)

Following diagnosis of an acquired neurological disability, spouses find themselves in situation where have to learn may new practical skills, be vigilant for their partner, and plan ahead. This is at a time when they have no previous experience, they are facing a new future, and facing changed relationships with partner, family and friends, and society at large. They often have to face these emotional changes alone, leading to a danger of feeling isolated and vulnerable. It is timely to consider whether health and social care professionals are a help or a hindrance to spouses.

The influence of health and social care professionals: help or hindrance?

Within the stroke study, spouses reported that they often gained relief within the hospital situation where their sense of being responsible for their partner was shared with staff. Mrs Curtis highlighted the value and support provided by the rehabilitation ward environment:

> Well [ward] was wonderful. I described it like going into a church. You know when you go into a church there is this wonderful feeling of peace and tranquillity, an aura, when you go into VH there is an aura of positiveness, of enthusiasm, it's a bit like a womb, didn't matter how depressed I was feeling I'd go there and I would enjoy my time there. (417/1)

Spouses took on responsibility for their partners' welfare from diagnosis onwards and while in hospital they felt they could make a direct contribution. In order to understand their present situation and plan for the future, spouses turned to health care staff for information. Spouses reported that they often felt frustrated that, although they felt they were the ones to organize the couples' future life, often information would be given to their partners, who either ignored it as they did not feel help was necessary or forgot to tell them. Often the staff who could give information were not easily available on the wards, or the appropriate member of staff was not identified. Spouses reported that they appreciated being invited to therapy sessions, so that they could be involved and 'see what was happening'. Overall spouses appeared to gain a limited understanding about the condition, daily care of their partner, or the implications for them in the future. Rosenthal *et al.* (1993), who explored the needs of 14 wives while their husbands were hospitalized following a stroke, concluded that the most important need was for information. They wanted to know what they could do to assist with care, to be involved in discharge planning, to know that their husband was well cared for, and to know what their husband would be able to do in the future. Although the spouses in the present study described great emotional changes, Rosenthal *et al.* found that that wives gave low priority to their own feelings. It appeared that in hospital wives were not ready, or did not have time, to reflect on their own needs.

The emotional situation of spouses and the effect of the information given did not always seem to be appreciated by the staff. Mrs Evans said:

> There were many times when they said little things, which made me really worried. (502/ 2)

Staff would mention something, which to them was apparent from their experience, but which came to spouses as a shock. When asked to describe these 'little things' Mrs Evans continued:

> Well it was just just little things. Like when A said that you know he'll probably never go back to work and you could have another stroke . . . I was grateful that he did give it to us straight but at the same time I was petrified that this was going to happen and could happen quite quickly you know. (513/1)

The difficulty of giving information in this situation was highlighted by Close and Proctor (1999). Due to the unpredictable nature of recovery it is difficult to give an accurate prediction of future and so replies tend to be vague. However Close and Proctor reported that relatives felt that staff did know but were not telling them. This creates a greater sense of isolation, as spouses felt that their views were not taken on board and that their concerns were not understood when they were already in a vulnerable position due to their worry for their partner.

While their partner was in hospital spouses reported that there was a sense that the stroke could be treated almost as an acute illness, that everything could be put on hold, and that things would get back to normal when their partner came home. Unfortunately this was rarely the case, Mrs Evans said looking back at six months:

> I think I thought once he came home everything was going to be fine again, and every-thing was positive and, and everything was going to move on. We put the [work]on hold, with the object of getting him on his feet and um, helping him as much as possible to feel that he was still part of life. But in fact it was bloody awful. (Laughs). I just came to a grinding stop. I couldn't cope. I couldn't cope with the emptiness around me, and I couldn't cope with D's helplessness. (48/2)

This is a reflection of the way chronic illness is treated within the present health care system that has an acute illness focus (Charmaz 1983; Strauss and Corbin 1988). Spouses equated hospitals with cure. Health care staff speak about recovery and their focus is short term and related to discharge (Pound and Ebrahim 1997), rather than seeing the hospital experience as the very first stage of a life-long change. The focus on short-term bodily and task-orientated improvement left little room for spouses to appreciate the longer term implications of their situation.

Individuals in a caring situation often take on their role without any choice, and often being unaware of the extent and nature of the caring responsibilities, and life changes they will be facing (Nolan and Grant 1992). As described above, there are many emotional consequences of their course of action. Often they are in their caring role before they have an opportunity to prepare for it. There is a large body of research to show that spouses are not given support in learning new skills for managing their new situation (McLean *et al.* 1991; Bunn 1996; Ward and Cavanagh 1997; Henwood 1998). The lack of support or recognition from health or social care staff may undermine spouses' already challenged sense of themselves and their future, as they have to learn by trial and error, and may have to live with a sense of failure.

While their partner was in hospital, spouses reported feeling tired, in a heightened emotional state with many worries and fears, and unresolved concerns. Very few described any process through which their own specific needs were addressed. If they were given any one-to-one attention from therapy staff, it was often to learn a practical skill such as helping their partner up from the floor if they fell. Mrs Curtis reflected on the time when her husband was in hospital and said:

> Everyone is Steven, Steven, Steven, Steven, Steven. The hospital is Steven, Steven, Steven, Steven, Steven. There's very very very little concern for the carer. No-one I mean I had to volunteer everything I said. Nobody sat me down and said, 'Now what are your circumstances? What are your conditions?'. I told people, because I needed help and so I volunteered the information. Nobody ever takes you by the hand and say's, 'How are you?'. (606/1)

This finding supports previous research, which has shown that if the needs of carers are assessed at all they are only considered near discharge and usually relate to the practical care of their family member (Waters and Luker 1996). Henwood (1998), in a survey of members of the UK National Carers Association, described how friends and family members are still marginalized by National Health Service staff. She found that hospital discharges were often poorly planned, and that often family and friends were left to cope with inadequate information and insufficient support. In a survey by Hedley (1996) of 216 younger UK Stroke Association members, 83% of carers reported that they did not feel adequately supported.

Why is it so difficult to support spouses? I would suggest that this is not because of individual health care staff, but because of the wider health care culture in which they are working. Spouses are seen as 'carers' and the use of the term carer has many wide implications that are not often recognized. When a person is defined as a carer they exist only in relation to the cared-for. They do not exist as a person in their own right with their own needs. Health care services are traditionally based on treating the individual ill body. The focus for professional intervention is the person who experiences the disability (Banks 1999; Heaton *et al.* 1999). Professionals are trained to accept a specific responsibility to one client or patient, whose interests are expected to prevail over those of others (General Medical Council 1995). Professionals are constrained in seeing spouses as a legitimate independent focus for service provision, and a spouse's claim on scarce resources is considered to be weaker than that of the 'patient'. Using present health models, it is seen as more legitimate to spend time with the stroke survivor, supporting them in improving their physical or self-care skills, than it is to discuss the emotional and practical needs of spouses in the new life situation in which they find themselves.

Because health care providers do not see it as their remit to offer a separate service to family and friends, spouses face additional challenges. In several studies family and friends have described how they had to resort to 'fighting' or 'pushing' for information as it was not freely volunteered (Godfrey and Moore 1996; Henwood 1998). This puts them in a difficult situation, as they do not want to be seen as pushy or selfish. Respondents in other studies have reported that they felt they were reneging on their responsibilities or failing in some way if they asked for help (Godfrey and Moore 1996; Ward and Cavanagh 1997). The position of family and friends is typified by the experience of a professional who became a carer and was herself passed around the system and given conflicting advice (Pitkeathley 1989). She said (p. 32):

> What amazed me most was how unwilling I was to make a fuss or get stroppy. I realised I felt I had no right to the services and I was asking for favours which somehow I had no right to.

Denman (1998) reported how one respondent found it difficult to ask about her husband once he was home, as the staff had been so friendly and she did not want to appear awkward or ungrateful for the care they had shown in hospital. Kautzmann (1993) highlighted that good knowledge leads to feelings of increased power and control within the home setting—the difficulty in accessing information puts spouses in a more powerless position.

There may also be a vicious circle. Pitkeathley (1989) suggested that lack of support for spouses may be compounded by health professionals' lack of confidence in addressing their needs. She suggested that health professionals may feel confident about making enquiries about physical aspects of care, as they could often offer an intervention such as providing a hand rail, but that they may be afraid to ask about psychological or social aspects of life, because they may feel they could not meet these needs. Bennett (1996) carried out a study to explore how nurses working on a stroke ward managed depression experienced by patients following a stroke. Nurses reported that they did not feel able to deal with the problem adequately. This was for two main reasons: the first was lack of time, the emphasis in service provision being on physical care; the second was a lack of knowledge about how to provide psychological support, as little training had been given. Physical care was divorced from psychological understanding.

Another limitation resulting from defining a spouse as a 'carer' is that the tasks involved in caring are personalized within one particular person—all responsibility is seen to focus on the one person. This reinforces the spouses' already keen sense of responsibility. Although there is increasing recognition that several people may be involved in the caring situation, one particular person—the 'primary caregiver'—is still highlighted as the focus of attention for health or social care intervention. As the role becomes personalized, the spouse may lose a sense of their own personhood and own rights as an individual. Spouses who identify closely with the role of carer may take on the dictionary definitions of being resilient, cheerful, *selfless*, and so limit their own life possibilities. The pattern and expectation that this sets up is reflected by Denman (1998), who reported that care is often provided by one family member and that a wider network is minimal or absent. Intervention becomes centred on the individual who is caring. This draws attention away from an analysis of the caring situation as a whole, to explore the physical social and emotional factors that could impact on the situation and that could be addressed.

The third, and probably the most fundamental, aspect of being defined as a carer is that when spouses are supported by health and social care professionals, they are supported to continue in their caring duties, rather than being seen as person in their own right who also has to live a life affected by chronic illness. By one year, the life of spouses in the stroke study had become subsumed to a caring role. The primary aim of rehabilitation is to improve the quality of life of the disabled person and to help them achieve their life goals. In this traditionally individualistic model, spouses are seen as agents to help the disabled person. Schumacher *et al.* (1998) typifies this overwhelming approach in the caring literature by noting that the aim of intervention is to help carers 'care well'. By defining spouses as carers, there are assumptions that spouses are primarily workers or contributors to the well-being of the cared-for. Spouses' own separate life goals, worries, or concerns are seen as secondary and they are rarely the focus of research or support.

Lack of acknowledgement by health care providers influences how spouses view themselves and their own health. Burton *et al.* (1997) found that spouses whose partners had daily care needs, paid little attention to their own physical well-being, such as taking adequate physical exercise, rest, and sleep, or taking themselves to their doctors. Nieboer *et al.* (1998) have recently concluded that activity restriction in 127 spousal caregivers of stroke, hip fracture, congestive heart failure, and myocardial infarction patients, could be seen as a critical mediator of an increase in their depressive symptoms. By supporting spouses in the subordinate position of being a carer, health care professionals may be contributing to future mental health problems.

Also while spouses become 'carers', their partners come to be seen as the 'cared-for' creating an impression of the passive victim, so denigrated by the disability movement (Swain *et al.* 1993). Health care interventions focus on bodily and task-based improvements of the disabled person, and wider life issues appear to be left to the spouse to organize. This expectation has far-reaching consequences; in the present study, although the majority of stroke partners had improved physically at one year (the majority were able to walk, a few had returned to driving), they were still being 'cared-for' by their spouses. They appeared to take a passive role within the relationship and main decisions appeared to be taken by the spouse. This would suggest that the stroke survivor was not supported to take a full role within the family or society.

Practical implications

When the experience of spouses of partners with acquired chronic neurological disability is seen in terms of identity change, rather than the traditional task-based or physical caring, new avenues for intervention become apparent. As the focus of concern is life change rather than just bodily change, spouses become a legitimate focus for attention in their own right. If using a life-narrative approach, the aim of the practitioner would be to help both the spouse and their partner live their own life with chronic illness.

This will require a sense that negotiation is essential between partners and that spouses do not automatically have to put their partners' needs before their own. This would reduce the chance of the following type of situation reported by Denman (1998). One of his respondents felt that, although he would be greatly helped if his wife went to day care, he reported that, 'It's got to be her idea to go, not mine. If I forced her to go I would be on a guilt trip for the rest of the day' (Denman 1998, p. 421). There would be recognition that a spouse, as well as their partner, has rights and responsibilities. It would be seen that both partners had to learn new practical skills and both partners in the couple would be given support to learn these skills.

By separating the concepts of spouses and the caring role, and considering 'spouses in a caring situation' rather than 'carers', the horizon of academics and practitioners can be broadened to consider two important aspects. First, that spouses are individuals with wider life opportunities beyond a caring role. Both partners of a couple could be supported in aiming for their own life goals within the framework of living with a chronic illness. Second, it would be recognized that spouses do not necessarily have to work within the caring situation alone, as the caring role would not be so closely bound to their identity. There would be recognition that caring situations are very complex and many differing interventions may be possible. For example, their disabled partner may be able to acquire more skills and confidence in managing alone, the physical environment could be adapted, and if identity and caring are separated, it may become more acceptable to spouses for other people to support their partner in the caring situation.

Also by focusing on identity, the experience of spouses in a caregiving situation is broadened to include the importance of 'being' as well as 'doing'. Secrest (2000) highlighted that it was important for nurses to 'be with' spouses, as well as doing things for them. The first step would be to recognize the huge emotional changes spouses are facing and to give them the opportunity to talk about their own life, worries, and concerns. From this chapter it can be seen that spouses may become very isolated and often have few opportunities to talk about their worries and fears with others. By listening, health and social care workers provide validation for the spouse's own experience, thus enhancing their sense of being a person in their own right. Also, and most importantly, the action taken by health and social care professional can be influenced by the thoughts and feelings of spouses, leading to a more collaborative and individual approach rather than intervention being based on clinical decisions alone. Kellett and Mannion (1999) have suggested that community nurses should foster an atmosphere of collaborative caring, through sharing perspectives, when they are considering their tasks and functions. Spouses living with stroke have proposed that any support needs to be ongoing (Denman 1998) due to the changing nature of their experience.

Summary

This chapter explores the experiences of spouses of partners with a chronic neurological illness. In order to gain a deeper understanding of their emotional experiences, a life-narrative approach has been used. This highlights the differences in how spouses see their past (before illness), their present, and their future life, and focuses on their sense of self. Three main conclusions are drawn. First, that spouses do see changes in themselves and their opportunities, which are often hidden from others. Second, that health and social care professionals may limit the spouse further by seeing them only in a caring role rather than a person their own right. Third, health and social care professionals may be able to address some of the emotional and practical problems experienced by spouses more effectively by considering the feelings and concerns of spouses before taking action.

References

Anderson, R. (1988). The quality of life of stroke patients and their carers. In *Living with chronic illness: the experience of patients and their families* (ed. R. Anderson and M. Bury), pp. 14–42. Unwin Hyman, London.

Anderson, R. (1992) *The aftermath of stroke: the experience of patients and their families.* Cambridge University Press.

Banks, P. (1999) *Carer support: time for a change of direction.* King's Fund, London.

Battista, J. and Almond, R. (1973). The development of meaning in life. *Psychiatry, 36,* 409–427.

Bennet, B. (1996). How nurses in a stroke rehabilitation attempt to meet the psychological needs of patients who become depressed following stroke. *Journal of Advanced Nursing, 23,* 314–321.

Bunn, F. (1996). The needs of families and carers of stroke patients. In *Stroke Services and Research* (ed. C. Wolfe, T. Rudd, and R. Beech), pp. 247–259. The Stroke Association, London.

Burton, L. C., Newsom, J. T., Schultz, R., Hirsch, C. H., and German, P. S. (1997). Preventative health behaviours among spousal caregivers. *Preventative Medicine, 26,* 162–169.

Bury, M. (1982). Chronic illness as biographical disruption. *Sociology of Health and Illness, 4,* 167–182.

Carter, J. H., Stewart, B. J., and Archbold, P. G. (1998). Living with a person who has Parkinson's disease: the spouse's perspective by stage of disease. *Movement Disorders, 13,* (1), 20–28.

Charmaz, K. (1983). Loss of self: a fundamental form of suffering in the chronically ill. *Sociology of Health and Illness, 5,* 168–195.

Charmaz, K. (1991). *Good days, bad days: the self in chronic illness and time.* Rutgers University Press, New Brunswick.

Close, H. and Proctor, S. (1999). Coping strategies used by hospitalised stroke patients: implications for continuity and management of care. *Journal of Advanced Nursing, 29,* (1), 138–144.

Conrad, P. (1987). The experience of illness: recent and new directions. *Research in the sociology of health care, 6,* 1–31.

Corbin, J. and Strauss, A. (1988). *Unending work and care.* Jossey Bass, San Francisco.

Cox, D. L. (1992). Perspectives of motor neurone disease. *Clinical Rehabilitation, 6,* 333–339.

Davis, L. and Grant, J. S. (1994). Constructing the reality of recovery: family home care management strategies. *Advanced Nursing Science, 17,* (2), 66–76.

Denman, A. (1998). Determining the needs of spouses caring for aphasic partners. *Disability and Rehabilitation, 20,* (11), 411–423.

Duijnstee, M. S. H. and Boeije, H. R. (1998). Home care by and for relatives of MS patients. *Journal of Neuroscience Nursing, 30,* (6), 356–360.

Ellis-Hill, C. S. (1998). *New world, new rules: life narratives and changes in self concept in the first year after stroke.* Unpublished PhD manuscript, University of Southampton.

Ellis-Hill, C. S, Payne S., and Ward, C. D. (2000). Self-body split: issues of identity in physical recovery following a stroke. *Disability and Rehabilitation. 22,* (16), 725–733.

Enterlante, T. and Kern, J. (1995). Wives reported role changes following a husband's stroke: a pilot study. *Rehabilitation Nurse, 20,* 155–160.

General Medical Council. (1995). *Duties of a doctor.* General Medical Council, London.

Gerhardt, U. (1990). Qualitative research on chronic illness: the issue and the story. *Social Science and Medicine, 30,* (11), 1149–1159.

Godfrey, M. and Moore, J. (1996). *Hospital discharge: user, carer and professional perspectives.* Nuffield Institute of Health, Leeds.

Goldstein, L. H. and Leigh, P. N. (1999). Motor neurone disease: a review of its emotional and cognitive consequences for patients and its impact on carers. *British Journal of Health Psychology, 4,* 193–208.

Grant, J. and Davis, L. (1997). Living with loss: the stroke family caregiver. *Journal of Family Nursing, 3,* (1), 36–56.

Habermann, B. (2000). Spousal perspective of Parkinson's disease in middle life. *Journal of Advanced Nursing, 31,* (6), 1409–1415.

Han, B. and Haley, W. E. (1999). Family caregiving for patients with stroke: review and analysis. *Stroke, 30,* 1478–1485.

Heaton, J., Arksey, H., and Sloper, P. (1999). Carers' experience of hospital discharge and continuing care in the community. *Health and Social Care in the Community, 7,* (2), 91–99.

Hedley, R. (1996). *Younger people have strokes too.* The Stroke Association, London.

Henwood, M. (1998). *Ignored and invisible? Carers experiences of the NHS.* Carers National Association, London.

Hill, C. S. (1997). Biographical disruption, narrative and identity in stroke: personal experience in acquired chronic illness. *Auto/Biography, 5,* 131–144.

Kautzman, A. N. (1993). Linking family and patient stories to caregivers; the use of clinical reasoning. *American Journal of Occupational Therapy, 47,* 169–173.

Kellet, U. M. and Mannion, J. (1999). Meaning in care: reconceptualizing the nurse-family carer relationship in community practice. *Journal of Advanced Nursing, 29,* (3), 697–703.

Kuyper, M. B. and Wester, F. (1998). In the shadow: the impact of chronic illness on the patients partner. *Qualitative Health Research, 8,* (2), 237–253.

McLean, J., Roper-Hall, A., Mayer, P., and Main, A. (1991). Service needs of stroke survivors and their informal carers: a pilot study. *Journal of Advanced Nursing, 16,* 559–564.

Morse, J. M. and Johnson, J. L. (1991). Towards a theory of illness. The illness constellation model. In *The illness experience: dimensions of suffering* (ed. J. M. Morse and J. L. Johnson), pp. 315–342. Sage, Newbury Park.

Nieboer, A. P., Schultz, R., Mathews, K. A., Scheier, M. F., Ormel, J., and Lindenberg, S. M. (1998). Spousal caregivers' activity restriction and depression: a model for changes over time. *Social Science and Medicine*, 47, (9), 1361–1371.

Nilsson, I., Jansson, L., and Norberg, A. (1997). To meet with a stroke: patients experiences and aspects seen through a screen of crises. *Journal of Advanced Nursing*, 25, 953–963.

Nolan, M. and Grant, G. (1992). Helping 'new carers' of the frail elderly patient: the challenge for nurses in acute care settings. *Journal of Clinical Nursing*, 1, 303–307.

Nolan, M., Grant, G., and Keady, J. (1996). *Understanding family care: a multidimensional model of caring and coping*. Open University Press, Buckingham.

Parker, G. (1993). *With this body: caring and disability in marriage*. Open University, Buckingham.

Parsons, T. (1951). *The social system*. Free Press, Glencoe.

Pitkeathley, J. (1989). *Its my duty, isn't it? The plight of carers in our society*. Souvenir Press, London.

Pound, P. and Ebrahim, S. (1997). Redefining 'doing something': health professionals' views on their role in the care of stroke patients. *Physiotherapy Research International*, 2, (2), 12–28.

Price, B. (1996). Illness careers: the chronic illness experience. *Journal of Advanced Nursing*, 24, 275–279.

Radley, A. (1994). *Making sense of illness—the social psychology of health and disease*. Sage, London.

Robinson, I. (1988). *Multiple sclerosis*. Routledge, London.

Robinson-Smith, G. and Mahoney, C. (1995). Coping and marital equilibrium after stroke. *Journal of Neuroscience Nursing*, 27, (2), 83–89.

Rolland, J. (1988). A conceptual model of chronic and life threatening illness and its impact on families. In *Chronic illness and disabilities* (ed. C. Chilman, E. Nunnally, and F. Cox), pp. 17–68. Sage, Beverley Hills CA.

Rolland, J. S. (1994). In sickness and in health: the impact of illness on couples' relationships. *Journal of Marital and Family Therapy*, 20, (4), 327–347.

Rosenthal, S., Pituch, M., Greninger, L., and Metress, E. (1993). Perceived needs of wives of stroke patients. *Rehabilitation Nursing*, 18, 148–167.

Schumacher, K. L., Stewart, B. J., Archbold, P. G, Dood, M. J., and Dibble, S. L (1998). Family caregiving skill: development of the concept. *Image: Journal of Nursing Scholarship*, 30, (1), 63–70.

Secrest, J. (2000) Transformation of the relationship: the experience of primary support persons of stroke survivors. *Rehabilitation Nursing*, 25, (3), 93–99.

Stewart, B. J., Archbold, P. G., Harvath, T. A., and Nkongho, N. O. (1993). Role acquisition in family caregivers of older people who have been discharged from hospital. In *Key aspects of caring for the chronically ill: hospital and home* (ed. S. G. Funk, E. H. Tornquist, M. T. Champagne, and R. A. Weise) pp. 25–47. Springer, New York.

Strauss, A. and Corbin, J. A. (1988). *Shaping a new health care system*. Jossey-Bass, London.

Swain, J., Finkelstein, V., French, S., and Oliver, M. (1993). *Disabling barriers-enabling environments*. Sage, London.

Vrabec, N. J. (1997). Literature review of social support and caregiver burden 1980–1995. *Image: Journal of Nursing Scholarship*, 29, 383–388.

Ward, H. and Cavanagh, J. (1997). A descriptive study of the self-perceived needs of carers for dependants with a range of long-term problems. *Journal of Public Health Medicine,* **19**, (3), 281–287.

Waters, K. R. and Luker, K. A. (1996). Staff perspectives on the role of the nursing rehabilitation wards for elderly people. *Journal of Clinical Nursing,* **5**, (2), 103–114.

Wellwood, I., Dennis, M., and Warlow, C. (1995). Patients and carers satisfaction with acute stroke management. *Age and Ageing,* **24**, 519–524.

Chapter 4

A longitudinal study of carers providing palliative care

Karen Rose

... it's a lot of hard work, this caring business. It is, yes. (Rose 1996, p.315)

So commented one of the informants in a longitudinal study of the experiences of informal carers of patients diagnosed with terminal cancer. The study, which took place between 1992 and 1996, was aimed not at assessing carers' needs or their satisfaction with support, but at gaining an understanding of what being a carer in this situation was like.

Informal caring is a growth industry in the United Kingdom. During the last census, it was estimated that there were approximately 6 000 000 adult caregivers in Britain (Office of Population Censuses and Surveys 1992). As the boundaries between formal and informal care, and nursing and social care become ever more blurred, with greater emphasis on home-based delivery of care for both acute and chronic conditions, the numbers of people expected to contribute at the informal level can only increase. These changes inevitably have implications for both informal carers, as they face a variety of demands on their time, and the nursing profession (Kirk and Glendinning 1998; Shyu 2000), including those providing palliative care.

Background

The original spur to carrying out the study on which this chapter draws was clinical contact, via patients suffering from incurable cancer, with family members involved in their care. However, it must also be remembered that such research studies are neither ahistorical nor acontextual, but are set in a particular time and place, of which the researcher must be aware (Giddens 1984). Before any fieldwork is commenced, adequate planning of the research strategy should take place, and a thorough literature review to locate the context of the work.

This chapter is intended to deal principally with what the experience of caring was like for carers of patients with incurable cancer and not to critique work already published on the subject. However, it is useful to have some understanding of the historical position of the study in relation to palliative cancer care research.

When preliminary work on the study began in 1992, there was already a large litera-ture available on informal caring but little of this was specifically about palliative cancer care. What there was stemmed chiefly from increasing interest in the process of grief and bereavement (Kubler Ross 1969; Parkes 1975), and the growth of the hospice movement in the latter part of the twentieth century. Early work tended to pay atten-tion to carers in respect of their relationship to patients. For example, a study by Hinton (1980) of 80 married patients dying of cancer showed that, whereas only 22 had discussed the possibility of dying with hospital staff, nearly twice as many (43) had spoken of this to their spouse. A longitudinal study by Stedeford (1981a, b), a hospice psychiatrist, identified the problems expressed by 41 terminally ill patients and their spouses. A quantitative approach was used and four key problem areas identified:

- unsatisfactory communication;

- the direct effects of the disease and its treatment;

- failure to adjust their lives to the changing circumstances;

- pre-existing marital and family problems.

Similar quantitative approaches were continued, as in a study by Swenson and Fuller (1992), which considered the experience of married couples where one partner had terminal cancer.

Research has also been conducted into the value of informal carers as reporters of patients' symptoms. Curtis and Fernsler (1989) found discrepancies between patient and carer accounts of pain, a finding supported by Higginson et al. (1994). The lat-ter also found similar discrepancies in patients' and carers' ratings of anxiety. How-ever, there was a significant degree of consensus as regards practical aid, wasted time, and communication. Field et al. (1995) found even less discrepancy between the accounts of carers and patients. In this study, no significant differences emerged between the two sets of reports on the patients' abilities to perform normal routines of daily living, their physical symptoms, or the care they received. In a more recent study, Hinton (1994) used both carers and patients to assess whether the home-care environment provided a satisfactory quality of life for these families. Like Field et al. (1995), he concludes that carers' and patients' reports are comparable, although unlike these researchers, he is assessing only psychological symptoms in both carers and patients.

Valuable as such data are, informal carers are not the focus of the research. Researchers began to recognize this and, by the late 1980s, studies started to appear that looked at carers' needs in palliative care. Hockley et al. (1988) showed that when carers are allowed to express what most concerns them personally, fear of caring for the patient at home is the problem most often identified. Jay (1990) drew attention to the importance of accurate assessment of relatives' needs to ensure adequate provi-sion of home services. Hull (1989) commented in a review article, that fear of not knowing what to do, together with not knowing what to expect, were two of the most potent sources of stress for carers.

Since the inception of the study discussed in this chapter, researchers have continued to pursue and enlarge upon these issues, in relation to carers as evaluators both of patients' quality of life (Sneeuw *et al.* 1997), and services provided to families where a member is suffering from terminal cancer (Fakhoury *et al.* 1996; Ingleton 1999; Jarrett *et al.* 1999). Both qualitative and quantitative methods have also been utilized to elucidate carers' concerns, needs, and experiences (Andershed and Ternestedt 1998; Payne *et al.* 1999). Indeed, the needs and experiences of families and informal carers of patients with terminal cancer are now an accepted part of the palliative care research repertory.

Method and informants

The brief literature review places the study to be presented here in its context. It is part of a continuum of research that seeks to help health care professionals to understand more fully what it is like to be an informal carer, and thereby to provide more sensitive and appropriate support (Rose *et al.* 1997; Rose 1998, 1999).

The intention of the study was to represent what it felt like to be providing palliative care at home to a relative. As this was therefore essentially a study about experience, a qualitative methodology was adopted, rooted in hermeneutic phenomenology (Heidegger 1962), and arguing that we can only understand human experience because we are human. Representing the experiences of informal carers was thus to be attempted by observing and interacting with their experience. A longitudinal strategy was adopted so that data could be collected over a period of time, acknowledging that people's feelings and perspectives on a situation fluctuate over time, and thus avoiding a 'snapshot' approach to the research question. In addition, it was felt that repeated contact with participants would allow the researcher to form more intimate relationships, which would yield richer data and allow the researcher to become more than simply an observer. Collins (1984) terms this participant comprehension, and this approach to the research relationship provided a practical expression of the Heideggerian theory underpinning the study.

The study took place in the north-west of England, with participants being accessed through a variety of sources, including district nurses, palliative care services, and religious leaders (Rose 2000). Data were collected from 21 primary carers (i.e. carers who had principal responsibility for the care of their loved one) and 11 secondary carers (i.e. carers who, although not the main carer, provided a substantial amount of support care). Families included in the study were either actively caring for a patient at time of first interview or were within one year of bereavement. Data were mainly collected through semi-structured, tape-recorded interviews conducted in the carers' homes. Ten telephone contacts and one written statement were included in data analysis, making a total of 55 informative interactions. Between one and four interviews took place with each informant.

In addition to the interviews, a triangulation strategy was also adopted by using a Mood Adjective Check List (Lishman 1972). This was initially intended to provide a quantitative adjunct to a qualitative study (between methods triangulation; Denzin 1970). However, it proved impossible to gain complete data sets, added to which participants tended to continue in interview mode and explore the meanings of the adjectives presented (Rose and Webb 1997); ultimately this provided valuable qualitative data from a different perspective and was therefore utilized as a form of within-method triangulation (Denzin 1970).

Whilst it would be false to claim that the sample of carers obtained was representative, the informants came from a variety of backgrounds (urban, suburban, and rural), from different socio-economic classes, ages, and sex. Wives were most commonly the carers, but husbands, adult children, children-in-law, and siblings were also well-represented. The experience of caring presented can therefore reasonably be supposed to reflect what it is like to a carer.

Data were analysed through repeated listening to tapes, and generation, comparison, and constant modification of themes emerging (Rose and Webb 1998). What shone through clearly time and time again in people's stories was the hard work involved for all the informants, whatever their background, and the immense impact that caring had on their lives.

Caring: work experience

The longitudinal strategy adopted, and the opportunity it afforded for developing relationships with the carers, resulted in an understanding that informal caring is not episodic, as is so much of formal caring, but the fabric of daily life. An entry in the reflexive journal kept during the conduct of the study demonstrates this realization (Rose 1996, p. 236):

> Reading some of the transcripts makes me think I've never understood what hard work really is. There's no real off-duty, half the time they don't know what they're dealing with or what to do. Added to that it's someone they love.

Reflecting on this entry generated the idea that the findings about what it was like to be a carer could be conceptualized under the heading of 'work', enabling the all-encompassing, time-consuming, and disruptive nature of the experience to be addressed from a number of different angles.

Caring: physical and emotional work

Caring is hard work both physically and emotionally. Attempting to separate these two factors creates an artificial division because one affects the other, thereby creating a total effect that is greater than the sum of its parts. For example, sleep disturbance has a physical effect and can also have psychological repercussions by increasing feelings of isolation.

In relation to practical care specifically, there was a wide range of need and a difference in the amount of physical help that individual patients required. What was common to nearly all carers was the experience of having to perform tasks to which they were unused and for which they could feel unprepared.

As a professional carer, it is easy to overlook the difficulties that informal carers may experience with basic nursing tasks, such as helping someone to dress, sit up in bed, wash, clean dentures or, as in the following extract, assist the patient to use a commode:

> That's something I don't think I'd ever like to do again, you know, putting a person on a commode. Oh, no. That was the worst thing even of all. The being sick, I coped with that, but putting a person on a commode and taking them off—that was something, oh, I hated.

Adding to the difficulty of carrying out a distasteful task was the knowledge that it would not be a single occurrence, but part of an ongoing situation:

> I've got to be here—I'm like the Prisoner of Zenda.

Performing the physical work of caring can also be made more difficult by the pre-existing relationship between the carer and patient. In the extract relating to use of the commode, quoted above, the relationship was that of daughter-in-law to father-in-law. Therefore, not only does the carer have the practical effort of helping the patient, and a feeling of revulsion for the job, but also the work of steeling herself to undertake an intimate task for a person who has always been held as a figure of some authority.

This example shows the kind of underlying pressures to which carers can be subjected. This is 'hidden' work of the type that writers such as Stanley (1987) and Star (1991) speak, and which is not immediately obvious to the casual observer. One of the informants, a man caring for his wife, summed this up when he spontaneously began an interview as follows:

> Yes. A lot of doctors don't understand. They can see you doing the physical bits and pieces, but they don't see the mental side—that's the worst side, you know. They can see you doing the washing, the ironing, the hoovering, cooking, all that. But the mental side, nobody sees that. That's the side I find very hard. I can cope with everything else, but the mental side, and the anguish and the frustration and temper that builds up, you've nowhere to release that—there's no outlet for that; it does become—well, it certainly does with me—a problem.

This feeling of being isolated and unable to let off emotional steam adds to the burden of 'hidden' work. Where no-one was available to whom carers could confide these feelings, no empathic listener who was felt truly to understand why they might feel these negative emotions, they often experienced feelings of guilt. Carers often felt that it was their job to be sympathetic and supportive to the patient, and felt guilty and ashamed when they could not maintain this facade the whole time:

> We had the odd blip, and I shall always feel guilty about that, but I can't change it.

Admitting such feelings can, in itself, be a stressful form of work, later in the interview, the same carer confessed:

> I've never told anyone about that before—you know, being so angry and shouting. I felt too ashamed.

This conversation took place several months after the patient's death, a fact that raises an important point: emotional work is a long drawn-out process, which continues well after the physical component of the caring experience is past.

Usual work

The physical work that carers perform is not exclusively connected to looking after the patient, they must also continue their usual work. The concept of 'usual work' is broad. It includes not only paid employment, but also other activities such as housework, shopping, maintaining the home, childcare, and outside commitments.

Amongst the primary carers who were still of working age, only one managed to combine the roles of carer and full-time worker and, in this case, it was through sheer necessity. The woman in question and her husband were farmers. As his illness progressed, she had to continue working or lose their livelihood. Her retrospective account of her experience shows just how difficult her situation was:

> Things just went from bad to worse, really. It was horrendous . . . Les wasn't there doing the farming and things were just going from bad to worse. . . . And having the worry of that as well, that was awful.

In the conflict between usual work and the work of caring, it should not be assumed that carers see their caring role as intrusive and disruptive, or that they do not want to care. This woman would have preferred freedom from other responsibilities so that she could devote herself to the caring role.

Where carers had given up work in order to devote themselves to looking after the patient, they rarely expressed any resentment directed at the patient. However, a number of problems were raised in relation to this situation. The informants in the study provided some evidence that employers were not always sympathetic, as this man's experiences show. He had needed time off work while his wife received active treatment. As her condition deteriorated, he needed more time off to look after her and their two children, aged sixteen and eleven:

> I went back in work and then I had to come off again. But work was all right apart from one bloke, wasn't he? He ignored me—the production manager at work. He ignored me because he didn't understand why I needed time off work . . . . He just totally ignored me—he didn't want to know . . . . That was his attitude . . . . He said, 'Well, I don't really understand'. And I said, 'You don't want to know, that's all. You're more interested in production and things like that'. He just wasn't interested.

As well as the potential problem of not being able to have absence from work sanctioned, carers' distress in this situation is heightened by feeling that employers do not care and simply do not want to understand the difficulties of the situation.

Sympathetic doctors can help carers to take time off work without loss of pay by signing them off as sick. One of the carers highlighted the potential difficulty this can cause. Her GP realized that she could not continue in her paid employment and provide full-time care for her relative, but also knew that loss of her earnings would have a serious impact on the family's finances. She therefore provided sick notes covering a period of several months, but attributed the need for leave to 'anxiety'. While this was helpful in the short term, in the longer term it could have detrimental effects on employment prospects because not all employers are sympathetic to a person who has had an extended period of sick leave for mental health problems.

Where carers were not supplied with sick notes and simply gave up work, this often had a profound financial effect, as this man's story shows:

> I mean, I finished work two and a half years ago because I used to work away and there was no way I could . . . . And you go from, like, earning £30 000 a year to nothing . . . .

'Going to nothing' had resulted in his having to sell a holiday home and live on the proceeds of the sale for some time until, eventually, the family were put in touch with a Macmillan nurse who told them about the various benefits to which they were entitled.

Financial difficulties undoubtedly add to an already distressing situation and the loss of usual, paid employment is a further problem. Loss of earnings, familiar work, and the companionship it affords have a profound effect on carers' quality of life:

> My married life's gone; my financial life's gone; your work life; your friends at work and that—you know, it's all gone. That's difficult to cope with.

This man's comments also show how the categories of experience are intimately linked to one another. Work affects not only time available for caring and finances, but also social relationships and a person's whole perception of self and position in society.

Other forms of usual work are the activities that go to make up everyday life, such as cooking, cleaning, shopping, minding grandchildren, which are all necessary and time-consuming and demand that carers juggle their lives to fulfil their caring role and meet the other demands on them. Despite the difficulty of managing competing demands, routine activities can be so much part of a carer's life that they do not want to stop doing them or may actually find the distraction and sense of normality they afford positively therapeutic, as this woman's comments show:

> [My sister] kept saying to me, 'For heaven's sake, sit down and stop!'. But, to me, as I said, carrying on and doing things—I didn't think then; otherwise, I would have brooded, think the worst or whatever .... But I'm all right ... because regarding the house, the garden, the shopping, the girls are offering. They've been a few times if the weather is bad for me, but I'd rather go and do it myself.

People who have always been independent and self-sufficient may not want to relinquish any of their usual work unless this becomes absolutely unavoidable, and may be using it as part of their coping strategy.

The working environment

'Environment' can mean the whole situation within which carers operate but, more obviously, it also means the setting within which their work is enacted. Although all the patients received in-patient care at some point, the environments that chiefly affected carers was the home and hospital out-patients settings.

Private homes are not designed as places where care of a sick person takes place. This affects the physical and emotional demands on carers. Seemingly simple tasks, like making sure that a patient upstairs in bed has adequate food and drink, necessitate someone having to go up and down stairs repeatedly. For older people especially, who may themselves not be entirely fit, this situation can present problems. Patients trying to maintain their independence in an unsuitable environment can also cause problems. Relatives often find it difficult to assert themselves in relation to patients, especially if the person has previously been something of an authoritarian figure to them. The following anecdote concerning a grandfather and granddaughter illustrates this:

She was going upstairs and he shouted, 'Don't come up, Jane. I'm in the bathroom, I've had an accident'. He'd had a bowel movement. She said to me that what he'd done when she finally did go up, he'd fell in the bathroom again (that was his second fall). She said, 'I heard the bang' and he shouted, 'Jane, you'll have to help me'. And she went up. He didn't have a stitch on the lower part. And, I mean, she is a quiet girl and it was her granddad—she must have been embarrassed.

In this case, the environment, the independence of the old man, the girl's relationship to him, and her inexperience as a nurse, all add to the difficulties of the situation.

Worrying about the patient and how the environment might affect him/her is also a common carer experience. For instance, one woman worried about her husband walking on his own, especially during chemotherapy treatment:

. . . because his leg hasn't been all so good, you see, while he was having the treatment. He's got arthritis in both legs. So, naturally you know, I like to be there, in case.

While relatively small in themselves, such considerations accumulate and are all part of the burden that carers carry.

In the home environment, even things designed to aid the carer can cause problems owing to lack of familiarity with equipment or, as in the following example, because carers are not always able to supervise the patient 24 hours a day:

He got a new electronic thing to lift the mattress up . . . instead of me having to lift him on my own, or me and my husband. He always said we hurt him, you see. I went out . . . he had the remote control, he had his water bottle, he had his tissues, he had a drink, everything at finger point. I went out and I was back two hours later . . . . The mattress was up to the highest point and he was across with his hands behind his head.

One of the most dispiriting aspects of providing informal care, which this story illustrates, was believing that you had done all you could to 'get it right' and finding out that the best laid plans came to nought.

Out-patient attendances for the majority of people in the study had been numerous; most cancer patients are treated for a long time and need out-patient appointments for a variety of reasons (e.g. radiotherapy, chemotherapy, follow-up). The potential drudgery of out-patient attendance was greatly alleviated by the attitude of staff. One woman commented on how friendly the staff were at a particular hospital, always remembering personal details and not treating people as a 'number', so that a visit there was seen:

. . . as home, really—it's like going in to see your doctor in the surgery.

The more formal the clinic, the more stressful attending it seemed. One patient had received a course of 18 treatments and a number of follow-up appointments, but his wife commented:

It was hard to get close to anyone. Not their fault. I was perhaps a bit overwhelmed by having to be there because it's a bit of a frightening hospital. People are treading on eggshells when they go there . . . . I don't think [he] saw the same doctor once.

Although this carer was not trying to find fault, it is important to realize the influence of continuity of care and a friendly atmosphere. Sensitivity on the part of out-patient staff made a far more positive contribution to out-patient attendance than the cosmetic appearance of buildings.

Related to these experiences, was that of perceived difficulty in obtaining access to an out-patient clinic. One woman recalled how her husband had been told by the surgeon that his cancer had returned and he was being referred to a radiotherapy clinic to be held the next week. The appointment did not arrive and the patient was in great pain. The carer had to call out her own doctor and district nurse and it took two phone calls from the GP before an appointment was finally sent. This placed a great strain on the carer because of having to see her husband suffer while apparently nothing was being done as promised. As she remarked:

> Waiting is the worst thing. When you know, you can deal with it in your own way.

Once again, the impact of staff actions is apparent. Patients and carers set great store by action occurring as promised.

Working relationships

The nature and closeness of particular relationships, and dealing with changed relationships, are intimately related to how carers perceive the caring experience. Carers' relationships with the patient, their relatives and friends can all be affected, first by the initial diagnosis of cancer, and later by its recurrence. A number of other factors are also influential in this respect:

- the various personalities involved;
- the pre-existing relationship;
- the effect of illness both physically and psychologically;
- the potential conflict that could arise because of a new and frightening situation.

For many carers, the most influential relationship was that with the patient. In the study, all the carers had a relationship of many years standing with the person for whom they were caring, and alteration of that was very difficult for them to come to terms with, whether in regard to physical or mental changes. One man summarized these feelings about his wife as follows:

> It's a different woman completely—a completely different person, mentally, physically and appearance; everything is changed.

He demonstrates an experience common to many carers: that loss of the person one knew and loved begins before death. This aspect of the experience is connected with the concept of anticipatory grief, beginning the grieving process while the patient is still alive but as the probability of death is ever more clearly accepted (Enlow 1986; Huber and Gibson 1990; Sweeting and Gilhooly 1990; Evans 1994); this was work of a very real sort for carers, which caused them much anguish, as they faced the diminishment of the person they had known:

> It was heart-breaking, because she was still my sister—but she wasn't.

Some carers found it hard to admit that any changes were taking place. When one patient, who had liver secondaries, commented that he thought he looked a bit yellow, his wife assured him that it was a suntan. It is possible to speculate that such pretences are not only for patients' benefit, but also a tacit denial on the part of carers as to the reality of what was happening, and which they did not, at that time, feel ready to address. Whatever the reason, such behaviour is likely to affect the relationship between carer and patient and to drive a wedge between them, making it impossible for them to deal with the situation as a team.

The degree to which relationships altered varied from one family to another, and was influenced by pre-existing personalities and roles. Some patients and carers realized that pre-existing roles would have to be modified in the light of the patient's impending death. This appeared to be beneficial to carers. For example, one woman expressed relief that her husband had explained to her about how to pay the rent and mow the lawn. Another carer was grateful that, before her death, his wife had shown him the basics of cooking and asked their daughter to ensure that 'Dad keeps up his standards'. At a post-bereavement interview, he appeared to be regarding this as a lifeline:

> And, you see, looking back, it's made me realize that she knew what was happening.

It almost seemed that her being able to assess the situation and take action about a practical matter before her death was now ensuring his continued well-being, both physically and emotionally.

At times, carers were forced by the demands of the illness to take on a new role in relation to the patient. An extreme example of this is that of the woman whose husband had a disfiguring facial cancer. From what she told me of their previous relationship, he had always looked after her. However, as his cancer progressed, it became increasingly embarrassing for him to go out, so that she was forced to take responsibility for paying bills, buying his clothes, and so on. Apart from the new role that she had to adopt, their relationship was further affected by the fact that he became increasingly bitter, frustrated and alienated from the world and from her. She found this emotional separation from her husband very hard to bear:

> One night he just got up, put his coat on and went out. He didn't say anything. He went like that. We didn't talk and we'd always been so close—it was awful.

This case provides a striking example of the way changes in physical appearance can affect the relationship between carer and patient. It is worth considering, however, that even less dramatic changes, often seen in cancer patients, such as weight loss, are all a reminder to the carer of the approach of death, and can therefore be distressing. Indeed, carers seemed to set great store by how the patient looked, equating appearance with the progress of the disease in the same way that Ferrell *et al.* (1991) suggest that they equate increasing pain with approaching death: if the patient looks well and is in no pain, the disease is thought to be in remission. It is important for professional carers to be aware of this because, while it is unkind to crush all hope, false expectations, on the basis of slim evidence, will ultimately result in disappointment and distress.

False hope on one side, opposed to realism on the other, can further affect the relationship between carer and patient, resulting in greater alienation and isolation. At one interview, a man, caring for his wife who had advanced cancer of the ovary, revealed that he was taking his wife to a health promotion course because he felt that if she could be kept optimally healthy in other ways, the cancer would stand less chance of progressing. The wife was present and, when he said this, smiled sadly, indicating that she knew the futility of what he was hoping might happen. The disparity in their response to the situation meant that rather than being able to provide mutual support, they were both dealing with the situation in isolation.

Certain relationships may have more potential for conflict inherent in them than others. This seemed to be the case in the women I interviewed who were, respectively, caring for an older sister and a father-in-law. The former acknowledged this herself:

> I always loved her, but it was very difficult for both of us . . . . And, with Amy being ten years older than I, she was always the older sister. No matter how old I was, I was still the little sister. And I think she found that quite hard because she always liked to be in control.

It is difficult to reverse the pattern of nearly 60 years where the person who was previously seen as the authoritative figure in the relationship now has to accept help from the 'junior'. How the relationship has previously been viewed by both carer and patient thus has implications for how it will be during the terminal phase.

Working companions: secondary carers

Carers' personal relationships were not, of course, limited exclusively to that with the patient, but also included their relationships with relatives and friends. Two scenarios emerged: either relatives and friends were extremely supportive and a good relationship was strengthened; or carers were left alone to their work and, consequently, felt increasingly isolated.

Where relatives and friends rallied round, they saw themselves very much as secondary carers or ancillary workers:

> We're all backing Alec while Alec looks after Sue.

> I'm here as a support for him, so that he's always got someone to turn to.

They were much more likely to provide emotional support and complementary help, performing separate tasks rather than assisting directly with tasks performed by the primary carer. Their input was highly rated by primary carers:

> I don't know what I'd do without my son and daughter. I know they're only a phone call away.

Much of the data obtained from secondary carers related to how they saw the situation as it affected the primary carer, rather than how it affected them personally. For example, a daughter remarked how many people concentrate on the patient and forget the strain on the main carer:

> But I think the carer gets left out because . . . it's all, 'How's Joe?' never 'How are you?'. And it's Mum that's doing all the work. Okay, he's had a major operation, but the carer's always the one that gets left out.

In another family, where the wife, the primary carer, had made light of her tasks, her daughter-in-law told me about the strain she felt was caused both emotionally and physically. She believed that this had resulted in the carer experiencing repeated episodes of vertigo and was worried about the ultimate outcome:

> My fear is that she will not last out, that something serious will happen to her, you know, and that she could, in fact, be the first one to die.

Such insights may have occurred because secondary carers could distance themselves, both physically and emotionally, from the situation. One such participant summed this up:

> But, it's alright for the family, Karen, isn't it? We can go home, we can leave, you know, Mum here, and we can go home. Go, but not forget, but go home and leave Mum here.

A degree of distance from the situation could be detected in certain topics that were addressed with much greater ease by secondary carers, notably the difficulty that unexpectedly prolonged survival could be:

> Originally, we delayed moving house, you see, because we saw Donald's consultant . . . and he said at that time (which is two years this autumn) he said six months to a year. So we . . . had that in mind, and it did go on so much longer than that. And I think I started to feel resentful . . . .

It is interesting to note how this secondary carer felt able to express a negative emotion and to discuss a very sensitive topic with a degree of detachment not encountered in primary carers.

Secondary carers not only provided a commentary on the caring situation, they were also an intimate part of it. Although many primary carers expressed great benefit from the input of secondary carers where they were present, in some circumstances a caring triad, as opposed to the more usual dyad, could precipitate conflict, with the patient playing one carer off against another. An example of this occurred during an interaction between a primary (wife) and secondary (daughter) carer:

> Wife: I just had to make him another sandwich. Yes, and he's got those drinks. You know, those like a meal . . . . The district nurse brought about a dozen in. He said, 'I'll have one of those', and you took him a sandwich up.
>
> Daughter: Bread and butter—he said that was all he wanted.
>
> Wife: He said, 'That's all she brought me up'.

Although this was not causing undue friction between the carers, such incidents have the potential to do so and, although the patient may not intend to cause extra work for the carer, this is effectively what happens.

Conflict also occurred in families where there was *potentially* more than one secondary carer. There were instances where secondary carers worked actively to complement one another's activities. For example, a son used to come round daily to entertain his father (the patient), while a daughter concentrated on supporting her mother (the carer). It was accepted by this family that a third sibling who lived in Northern Ireland could, in the main, offer only emotional support. However, inequality of sibling support could cause tension, as in the case where two sisters felt that a geographically nearer sister was not giving as much support as might have been expected. It is always important to be aware of family dynamics, and to identify areas where, even in close, supportive families, conflict can arise that may have implications for professional support workers.

Working ethics

Although for some informants caring for their relative was something that 'just happened' and they simply got on with the practicalities, others commented more abstractly about the meaning of being a carer, raising points about the ethical basis of the role they were adopting, and discussing the reasons why they felt they should undertake the task. Essentially, the ethical basis for caring consisted of three components: love, duty, and promising, either singly or in combination. For example, one informant, who cared for his wife, clearly felt it was his duty:

> Well, it's something you just do. Don't get me wrong—it's not something I want to do, but it's got to be done. Somebody's got to do it. I couldn't turn my back on the lady.

Another said:

> So, there was no question. My wife was ill and I'll do my best to look after her . . . . I just thought 'Right, we've been together 50 years and I made a promise,' and tried to carry it out to the best of my ability.

One man, speaking of how difficult he found the caring role, emphasized the importance of his marriage vows in taking on the care of his wife, but felt that his love for her was an equal source of motivation:

> But you don't think of these things when it's for love, do you?

Ethical issues did not only encompass the reasons why people were acting as carers, but also their behaviour within the caring role. Some carers spoke of the need to act as the patients' advocate in ensuring that they received appropriate treatment at the appropriate time. This included fighting to get appointments at hospitals, initiating introduction to the Macmillan service, pressing for information about financial help, and challenging a GP who was unhappy about prescribing an expensive treatment recommended by the hospital. While carers were not resentful for themselves about having to act as advocates in this way, they were concerned by the fact that it was often so difficult to obtain something which they felt was vital to the patients' well-being. This woman spoke of the difficulty she had experienced in obtaining support on two separate occasions: first, when her mother had been terminally ill with cancer of the bowel; and, more recently, when her husband was given a similar diagnosis:

> On both occasions I felt that there could have been some liaison between the hospital and the Macmillan nurses . . . . I mean, we got it, but we had to go out searching for it.

These more assertive carers were often also worried about the level of support and care likely to be forthcoming for those who were less able to speak up for their needs and rights. As one patient remarked to his wife who had repeatedly acted as his advocate:

> Not everybody's got a wife that can do it or will do it.

The importance of incidents such as these, as well as demonstrating an ethical belief held by carers, lies in the way it indicates the aloneness to which carers and patients are sometimes subjected, a feeling that is exacerbated by the perceived difficulty of gaining any control over the situation. In the instances I have cited, carers obviously perceived the need to *fight*, not even negotiate, for what they believed to be the right course of action. At a time of distress, it is an indictment of professional services and communications that carers felt that the responsibility to speak up for patients' rights was theirs, rather than an informal, collective decision made by all parties concerned.

Closely related to ethical issues were the religious and spiritual components of caring. The belief systems of the informants varied greatly, and not all of them addressed these issues in any depth, but several remarked on the degree of help they had received from spiritual sources. Regardless of religious affiliation, carers indulged in metaphysical speculation about the situation and often expressed a mixture of religious belief and disbelief:

> I can't see how religion can come into it, when I've got to see Joe suffer in the end . . . . No, I don't disbelieve, but when you get somebody like that, like Joe, and you think, 'Why is God making him suffer like he's going to?'. Oh, as I say, there's thousands like him, I know, but I think this is a time when God's trying you out to see if you can—you know what I mean? These things are sent to try us, aren't they? And this is my trying time.

Both carers who practised a faith and those who did not grappled with questions about why their relative had developed the illness and what it meant; such abstract considerations were not confined to those who either did, or did not, profess a religious belief. However, those with a faith did sometimes seem to find benefit in religious practice. These people mentioned especially drawing comfort from prayer, as in this instance:

> I always feel better when I've been to church and said some prayers, or wherever I've said some prayers—you always feel that bit better, don't you? Feel as if you've got some sort of support.

The value of prayer was not felt only at an individual level. Prayerful activity by others was also seen as supportive as this exchange between a husband and wife shows:

> Husband: Well, we've had Roman Catholics saying masses, Islamic friends praying for us, a Buddhist friend...she said a mantra . . . . It shows really the identity of the spiritual—all these people are on their own path and they're all supportive.

> Wife: It's like good 'vibes', really. And people are praying and thinking good thoughts on your behalf. I'm sure that it must produce a good energy somehow.

Religious leaders themselves were significant in this respect. As with other professionals, it was their attitude that was seen as most crucial; being friendly, accessible, and non-judgemental, whilst unobtrusively offering appropriate support could be very valuable. For instance, one woman told how a rabbi and his wife had spent the night with her to offer practical help when her husband was dying. Another recounted how her husband, a lapsed Catholic, had been twice divorced before marrying her. She was an agnostic, but was happy to arrange for a priest to visit when her husband requested this. What she was not prepared for the attitude of the priest:

> . . . the priest was absolutely lovely, popped in every day . . . and this lovely priest took it all in his stride and I think he'd probably have married us, if we'd asked him, you know. He was quite happy to give Alan complete absolution, no fuss. And that was an enormous comfort . . . .

The result of the priest's handling the situation sensitively was that the patient received spiritual comfort and the carer felt better because she knew that the priest had been able to help her husband.

Failure to behave in an appropriately supportive way and simply utter platitudes, as happened to a couple in their forties where the wife was terminally ill, is not helpful:

> We had a word with [the priest]. He just sat down. He said, 'Don't let it get you down'.

How can professionals help?

This chapter has been intended to give an insight into the everyday worlds of people who are caring for a relative dying of cancer, and not to prescribe how professionals should deal with this group. However, insights are useless if they are not translated into practice. Each patient and each carer is an individual and will require different types and degrees of support. In all cases, the right approach will, however, yield benefits; it can be summarized under the headings of communication, collaboration, commitment, consistency, confidence, consideration, control, and context:

1 *Communication*: it is essential for professionals to maintain good communication amongst themselves, between themselves and informal carers and to facilitate communication between carer and patient.

2 *Collaboration*: the *minimum* aim of professionals in this respect should be to ensure that carers are not treated only as resources. Carers need to feel that they are not working alone, but that there is someone there working alongside them.

3 *Commitment*: carers need to be sure that support once offered is fully committed to the end.

4 *Consistency*: carers develop relationships with people whom they see on a regular basis; they need to be confident that the same person will always be available, so that receiving conflicting advice from a variety of sources is avoided.

5 *Confidence*: practitioners owe it to the families with whom they work to maintain a high standard of knowledge so that confidence in their management and advice is justified.

6 *Consideration*: consideration of people as people at an individual level, with individual needs, is likely to foster appropriate attitudes and assistance in each family.

7 *Control*: this implies finding the right balance, so that carers feel that they are receiving help from someone who understands, but are not overwhelmed by the situation, while at the same time respecting the key role that the informal carer occupies.

8 *Context*: nurses working with families facing terminal illness must have an awareness of the context within which the care is taking place. Such an awareness implies not only an understanding of the immediate environment, but an ability to work with informal carers as part of the caring team within that environment. At the same time, this must be done with a due awareness of the availability of, and constraints on, resources.

Condensing the implications for professional practice in this way does not imply that there is a simple way of dealing with informal carers of terminally ill cancer patients or that professionals should merely follow a checklist of interventions. If we do this, we are potentially guilty of the kind of diagnostic reductionism which Holden (1990) argues is not the fault of a particular model of care, but of the people who implement the model insensitively. Above all, it is necessary to be sensitive to each carer and to assess the needs of each family individually, always bearing in mind that those actually involved in caring are in possession of the most detailed and expert knowledge about their needs (Keady and Nolan 1994).

Concluding remarks

The concept of a job of work has been employed to elucidate the complex and difficult experience of caring. It is work that has practical and emotional components and, like any job, is affected by co-workers, personal abilities, level of knowledge, and degree of support to the main worker. Frequently, the experience has been presented in negative terms. This reflects how the carers related their stories, emphasizing what a lonely and isolating experience informal caring can be. However, caring is not an entirely negative experience and although it is undoubtedly stressful, the carers represented here did, at times, find satisfaction in their roles as other studies have shown (Dawson 1991; Grant and Nolan 1993). One woman, for instance, when completing the questionnaire, came to the word 'unhappy' and said:

> 'Unhappy?' Yes, but happy about what we'd got. I mean, once we found out what we were dealing with, we had some happy times. Sad—but definitely made the most of the situation.

Comments such as this and the stories that some carers told about how they and the patients achieved goals, organized parties, holidays, and outings with, and for, the patient, which gave all concerned pleasure, indicate that it is possible to find satisfaction, and a degree of happiness, in the caring experience.

References

Andershed, B. and Ternestedt, B-M. (1998). Involvement of relatives in the care of the dying in different care cultures: Involvement in the dark or in the light? *Cancer Nursing*, 21, (2), 106–116.

Collins, H. M. (1984). Researching spoon-bending: concepts and practice of participatory fieldwork. In *Social researching: politics, problems, practice* (ed C. Bell and H. Roberts), Ch.3. Routledge and Keegan Paul, London.

Curtis, A. E. and Fernsler, J. I. (1989). Quality of life of oncology hospice patients; a comparison of patient and primary caregiver reports. *Oncology Nursing Forum*, 16, (1), 49–53.

Dawson, N. J. (1991). Need satisfaction in terminal care settings. *Social Sciences & Medicine*, 32, 1, 83–87.

Denzin, N. K. (1970). Strategies of multiple triangulation. In *The research act: a theoretical introduction to sociological methods*, Ch.12. Aldine, Chicago.

Enlow, P. M. (1986). Coping with anticipatory grief . . . catharsis of an anguished daughter. *Journal of Gerontological Nursing*, 12, (7), 36–37.

Evans, A. (1994). Anticipatory grief: a theoretical challenge. *Palliative Medicine*, 8, (2), 159–165.

Fakhoury, W. K. H., McCarthy, M., and Addington-Hall, J. M. (1996). Which informal carers are most satisfied with services for dying cancer patients? *European Journal of Public Health*, 6, (3), 181–187.

Ferrell, B. R., Cohen, M. Z., Rhiner, M., and Rozek, A. (1991). Pain as a metaphor for illness—Part II: Family caregivers' management of pain. *Oncology Nursing Forum*, 18, (8),1315–1321.

Field, D., Douglas, C., Jagger, C., and Dand, P. (1995). Terminal illness: views of patients and their lay carers. *Palliative Medicine*, 9, (1), 45–54.

Giddens, A. (1984). *The construction of society.* Polity, Cambridge.

Grant, G. and Nolan, M. (1993). Informal carers' sources and concomitants of satisfaction. *Health, Social Care & Community*, 1, (3),147–159.

Heidegger, M. (1962). *Being and time* (trans. J. Macquarrie and E. Robinson). Harper and Brothers, New York.

Higginson, I., Priest, P., and McCarthy, M. (1994). Are bereaved family members a valid proxy for a patient's assessment of dying? *Social Science Medicine*, 38, (4),553–7.

Hinton, J. (1980). Whom do dying patients tell? *British Medical Journal*, 281, 1328–1330.

Hinton. J. (1994). Can home care maintain an acceptable quality of life for patients with terminal cancer and their relatives? *Palliative Medicine*, 8, (3), 183–196.

Hockley, J. M., Dunlop, R., and Davies, R.J. (1988). Survey of distressing symptoms in dying patients and their families in hospital and the response to a symptom control team. *British Medical Journal*, 296, 1715–1717.

Holden, R. J. (1990). Models, muddles and medicine. *International Journal of Nursing Studies*, 27, (3), 223–224.

Huber, R. and Gibson, J. (1990). New evidence for anticipatory grief. *Hospice Journal*, 6, (1), 49–67.

Hull. M. M. (1989). Family needs and supportive nursing behaviours during terminal cancer: a review. *Oncology Nursing Forum*, 16, (6), 787–792.

Ingleton, C. (1999). Service evaluation. The views of patients and carers on one palliative care service. *International Journal of Palliative Nursing*, 5, (4), 187–195.

Jarrett, N. J., Payne, S. A., and Wiles, R. A. (1999). Terminally ill patients' and lay-carers perceptions and experiences of community-based services. *Journal of Advanced Nursing*, 29, (2), 476–483.

Jay, P. (1990). Relatives caring for the terminally ill. *Nursing Standard*, 5, (5), 30–32.

Keady, J. and Nolan, M. (1994). The carer-led assessment process (CLASP): a framework for the assessment of need in dementia caregivers. *Journal of Clinical Nursing*, 3, (2), 103–108.

Kirk, S. and Glendinning, C. (1998). Trends in community care and patient participation: implications for the roles of informal carers and community nurses in the United Kingdom. *Journal of Advanced Nursing*, 28, (2), 370–381.

Kubler-Ross, E. (1969). *On death and dying*. Macmillan, New York.

Lishman, W. A. (1972) 'Selective factors in memory. Part 2: affective disorders'. *Psychological Medicine*, 2, 248–253.

Office of Population Censuses and Surveys. (1992). *General Household survey: carers in 1990*. HMSO, London.

Parkes, C.M. (1975). *Bereavement: studies of grief in adult life*. Penguin, Harmondsworth.

Payne, S., Smith, P., and Dean, S. (1999). Identifying the concerns of informal carers in palliative care. *Palliative Medicine*, 13, (1), 37–44.

Rose, K. E. (1996). *Nursing a dying relative: the experience of informal carers of terminally ill cancer patients*. Unpublished PhD thesis, University of Manchester.

Rose, K. E. (1998). Perceptions related to time in a qualitative study of informal carers of terminally ill cancer patients. *Journal of Clinical Nursing*, 7, (4), 343–350.

Rose, K. E. (1999). A qualitative analysis of the information needs of informal carers of terminally ill cancer patients. *Journal of Clinical Nursing*, 8, (1), 81–88.

Rose, K. E. (2000). Gaining access to potential research participants. *Professional Nurse*, 15, (7), 465–467.

Rose, K. E. and Webb, C. (1997). Triangulation of data collection: practicalities and problems in a study of informal carers of terminally ill cancer patients. *Nursing Times Research*, 2, (2), 108–116.

Rose, K. E. and Webb, C. (1998). Analyzing data: maintaining rigor in a qualitative study. *Qualitative Health Research*, 8, (4), 556–562.

Rose, K. E., Webb, C., and Waters, K. (1997), Coping strategies employed by informal carers of terminally ill cancer patients. *Journal of Cancer Nursing*, 1, (3), 126–133.

Shyu, Y-I. L. (2000) Patterns of caregiving when family caregivers face competing needs. *Journal of Advanced Nursing*, 31, (1), 35–43.

Sneeuw, C., Aaronson, N. K., Sprangers, M. A., Detmar, S. B., Wever, L. D., and Schornagel, J. H. (1997). Value of caregiver ratings in evaluating the quality of life of patients with cancer. *Journal of Clinical Oncology*, 15, (3), 1206–1217.

Stanley, L. (1987). Some notes on 'hidden' work in public places: the case of Rochdale. In *Essays on Women's Work and Leisure and 'Hidden' Work*. Studies in Sexual Politics 18: Department of Sociology, University of Manchester.

Star, S. L. (1991). The sociology of the invisible: the primacy of work in the writings of Anselm Strauss. In *Social organization and social processes:essays in honor of Anselm Strauss*. (ed. D. Maines). Hawthorne, NY: Aldine de Gruyter. (Manuscript courtesy of the author).

Stedeford, A. (1981a). Couples facing death: I-psychosocial aspects. *British Medicine Journal,* **283**, 1033–1036.

Stedeford, A. (1981b). Couples facing death: II-unsatisfactory communication. *British Medicine Journal,* **283**, 1098–1101.

Sweeting, H. N. and Gilhooly, M. L. M. (1990). Anticipatory grief: a review. *Social Science & Medicine,* **30**, (10), 1073–1080.

Swenson, C. H. and Fuller, S. R. (1992). Expressions of love, marriage problems, commitment, and anticipatory grief in the marriages of cancer patients. *Journal of Marriage & The Family,* **54**, (1), 191–196.

Chapter 5

Who is a carer? Experiences of family caregivers in palliative care

Paula Smith

Introduction

With increasing numbers of terminally ill people remaining at home (Seale and Cartwright 1994), family caregiving is an important aspect of palliative care. Since the inception of the modern hospice movement there has always been a strong emphasis on support for the family of the terminally ill person (Seale 1989), however, there is little clear understanding of how this might be achieved. Furthermore, the emphasis of supporting the family implicitly assumes that they will be willingly involved in the situation and able to undertake some form of support for the ill person themselves.

This chapter will explore the experiences of a selection of individuals who were giving care to a family member with a terminal diagnosis of cancer, and who were in receipt of specialist palliative care services (SPCS). The chapter is based on one area of analysis from a research study that explored the perceptions of family caregivers' within palliative care. Specifically this chapter will explore the family caregivers' perception of their role and their relationship with visiting health professionals.

The study on which this chapter is based originated as a result of my professional background working with both patients and families of individuals who had a terminal diagnosis of cancer. I often found that a large part of my time was spent supporting family members, and my desire was to better understand their perception of the situation in order to be able to provide more effective care and support.

An initial literature search revealed that whilst there was an abundance of literature on 'carers', there was very little that related specifically to those in a palliative care setting. Although there may be many similarities between carers of different groups, a particular disease trajectory and the certain process of dying acknowledged within palliative care may have an impact on the situation that can not be accounted for in the general literature. Prior to presenting the findings I shall briefly review some of the literature that influenced the structure of the study.

Background

Increasingly, family caregivers are being relied on to provide support and care for members of their immediate family (Clark 1995; Heaton 1999). Within palliative care there has been little discussion about the nature of the family caregiving role or the perception that family caregivers themselves may have about their involvement in caring for the ill person. Understanding the needs and perceptions of this group is important as improved treatment regimes and symptom control have resulted in palliative care being increasingly undertaken at home. Up to 90% of patients now spend the majority of their last year of life at home (Seale and Cartwright 1994). This places pressure on the family and immediate kin who are often referred to as the informal or family 'carer'. Whilst remaining at home is often the preferred place for both patient and their family (Thorpe 1993), one reason for admission to a hospice or hospital is a breakdown in this caring network (Addington-Hall *et al.* 1991).

The question remains who is a carer, and what is their position in palliative care? The term carer was not used until the 1970s (Heaton 1999), and Twigg *et al.* (1990) suggest it stems from a service orientation and was originally intended to reflect the work undertaken by professional or formal carers. Informal carers, on the other hand, are generally unpaid and untrained, and provide care as the result of a pre-existing relationship with the cared for person. Informal carers are also referred to as family caregivers, lay carers, home carers, and unpaid or untrained carers. The distinction between the two terms surrounding training and expertise implies that formal or professional care is more desirable than informal or unpaid care. However, this fails to take account of the acquired experience and expertise developed by informal carers, particularly if they have been caring for a long time (Nolan *et al.* 1996). Heaton (1999) argues that more recently there has been a polarization of informal and formal roles in social policy that has conceptualized the informal carer as the primary provider of care in the community and formal care as a sustainor of this informal network.

Despite an explosion in the literature surrounding informal care, definitions of the term 'carer' remain ambiguous (Twigg 1989; Spackman 1991). Although there is some acknowledgement that a carer will be supporting another person in some way (Pitkeathley 1989; Neale and Clark 1992; The Carers National Association 1996), the extent, level, and degree of such support is unclear. Few of the definitions focus on the understanding and perception of the individual carer, and those that do tend to concentrate on the negative rather than the positive aspects of the role.

As women have traditionally assumed the role of family caregiver, Neale and Clark (1992) suggest that such care is closely bound to family obligation and perceptions surrounding the woman's role. Arber and Gilbert (1989), however, highlighted the large numbers of men who participate in caring, particularly if they are the spouse of the cared for person. In addition, elderly men and women have been found to provide equal amounts of co-resident care, which suggests that there are few gender inequalities amongst older spouses (Arber and Ginn 1990).

Although each family structure and organization is different, societal norms and obligations do affect the conduct of family members. Within the UK, there has been increasing pressure on families to provide care for sick or disabled members within the community (Clark 1995; Heaton 1999). Individual expectations within the family also affect the degree to which the family caregiving will be expressed. A sense of obligation and duty to their family members is a strong motivation for caregiving if someone is diagnosed with a chronic illness or disability. Likewise, reciprocity for actual or anticipated need is a factor in an individual's decision to become a family caregiver (Neufeld and Harrison 1998).

Family caregivers' perceptions of palliative care have, until recently, been limited to them acting as a proxy for patient satisfactions with services (Field 1995; Nekolaichuk *et al.* 1999). Some studies have explored the family caregivers' experience of burden (Theis and Deitrick 1987; Carey *et al.* 1991; Hinton 1994; Addington-Hall and McCarthy 1995), which has failed to recognize the positive aspects to the caring role (Nolan *et al.* 1995).

More recently, a number of studies (Duke 1998; Rose 1998, 1999) have begun to explore the experience of family caregiving within palliative care. However, there remains little evidence of how family caregivers perceive the role of 'carer' or their relationship with health professionals. The current study therefore aimed to identify how family 'carers' perceived their role in a palliative care setting, and sought to explore the nature of their relationship with visiting health professionals.

Method and participants

In order to explore the dynamic and changing nature of caring for a family member in a palliative care setting, it was decided to undertake a longitudinal study. The study was based on an approach described by Yin (1994), case study research, which is a comprehensive strategy encompassing design, data collection, and data analysis, and which allows the contextual information surrounding a situation to be explored.

Sixteen family caregivers (eight male and eight female) participated in the study. The men were all husbands of the patients. Six women were wives of the patient and two were adult daughters. The age range of the family caregivers was 37–77 with a mean of 56.8 years. All were recruited from two areas in the south of England and were identified by the visiting Macmillan or home care nurse. The family caregivers were looking after someone who had a diagnosis of cancer and a prognosis of six months or less. All the names of the participants have been changed to protect their identity, instead pseudonyms have been used to maintain the contextual feel of the data and quotes provided.

Each family caregiver was visited up to four times over a 4-month period. Wherever possible, family caregivers were interviewed alone, although seven chose to be interviewed with the person they were caring for. Both a semi-structured interview and a number of standardized measures of caregiver activity, stress, and social support were administered. In this chapter I will draw on accounts provided by the family caregivers during interviews. All interviews took place in the caregiver's own home, and lasted between one and two and a half hours.

Each interview was tape recorded and later fully transcribed. Each transcript was then subjected to continuous reading and re-reading in order to elicit themes and issues that were relevant to the family caregivers. During this process it became clear that identification with the term 'carer' was variable. Six family caregivers readily identified with the term, whilst the remainder did not. This had implications for the family caregivers interaction with the health professionals with whom they came into contact, and it is these issues that I wish to explore in this chapter

The family caregivers

It was clear from the interviews with the family caregivers that each had a different and particularly personal interpretation of their own situation. However, a full understanding of the family caregiver's perspective would not be possible without taking into account the often complex and dynamic caregiving relationship that had developed between the family caregiver, the ill person, and others involved in the situation.

Identifying with the term 'carer'

Only six (one male and five female) family caregivers readily identified themselves as a 'carer' to their loved one. All of these individuals had been giving care for well over a year and in some cases for a number of years, especially if the person they were caring for had a chronic illness or disability prior to a cancer diagnosis. Both daughters in the study identified themselves as a carer for their mothers.

For some family caregivers there appeared to be a pattern of caring throughout their lives, which could be thought of as a 'caring career'. For these individuals large parts of their adult life, and sometimes childhood, had been spent caring for others, particularly close kin. For example, Mrs Vaughan who was 52 years old and caring for her husband of 31 years. He had a very disfiguring facial carcinoma that had been originally diagnosed 4 years previously. They lived together in their own home, and were both fully aware of the husband's diagnosis. Mrs Vaughan had expressed a desire to know as much as possible about the prognosis of her husband's condition.

Mrs Vaughan had one married son who lived approximately 8 miles away, and with whom they had little contact due to his shift work as a paramedic. Mrs Vaughan was also the primary family caregiver for her mother who had Parkinson's disease, and visited her every day to prepare meals and attend to her financial affairs. Mrs Vaughan had a very supportive neighbour living next door, who occasionally sat with her husband so that she could go shopping. Mrs Vaughan's own health was generally poor and she felt caring for her husband had exacerbated this.

Mrs Vaughan identified strongly with the term 'carer', and was an active member of the local carers support group. She had even written articles in the local paper about her life as a carer. Mrs Vaughan suggested her role as a carer began as a small child when she had been involved in caring for her grandmother's emotional well being:

> I didn't actually do the nursing, but I was there to give her security.

This pattern had continued throughout her life, as she willingly, and apparently actively, sought a caring role first for elderly neighbours, and then her own mother and husband:

> I've always done something for somebody.

Clearly Mrs Vaughan gained a lot of personal satisfaction and pleasure from the role of carer, and was very proud of her achievements. For Mrs Vaughan, being a carer was not necessarily tied up with having received formal training, but was inherited. For this reason Mrs Vaughan believed that there were 'natural carers':

> It stems from the family because we've got a lot of medical professional people in our family, so it's born in, it's in your genes . . . . Some people are natural carers some people aren't.

A large part of Mrs. Vaughan's sense of identity was associated with the role of carer, and she described her biggest worry as knowing what she would do when her caring role ended:

> What do the carers do when the caring ends?

Such a strong identity with a caregiving role could have serious implications for an individual following bereavement, where there would not only be a loss of the cared-for person but also the role to which there was attached a clear sense of purpose and usefulness. Assisting family caregivers who identify with the term carer in this way to adjust to the multiple losses that will occur following bereavement may be a useful area for development of bereavement services within palliative care.

For other family caregivers who identified with the term carer this had occurred as they came into increasing contact with health and social care professionals. Mrs Page was 58 years old and caring for her mother who lived in the next street. She lived with her husband, who had taken early retirement due to ill health, and had two daughters, who both lived locally, and one son, who lived approximately 100 miles away. Mrs Page also had two brothers, both living a long distance away and who were therefore unable to contribute to the day to day care of their mother.

Mrs Page generally reported few problems with her own health but did feel extremely 'run down' and 'up tight'. For Mrs Page this may have been partly due to the extended period of caring for her mother, which had begun 4 years earlier on the death of her father and had intensified since her mothers diagnosis with cancer 1 year previously. Furthermore, she sometimes felt torn between caring for her mother and her responsibilities towards her own husband and children, and work commitments.

Although Mrs Page did not assist her mother with personal care or general household tasks, she was responsible for all the practical and emotional support of her mother and, in particular, her medication. Mrs Page had learnt to acknowledge her role as carer only when she had been called a carer by a member of the social services day-care centre that her mother attended weekly:

> And she said to me 'You must be your mother's carer'. So I thought, well I suppose I am.

For Mrs Page, development of a carer identity was strongly influenced by her interactions with others, as prior to this experience Mrs Page had not considered herself to be a carer but a daughter.

Kinship, obligation, and reciprocity

For the majority of the family caregivers, however, they perceived their position to be more strongly related to their relationship with the ill person rather than a particular role or job. Indeed much of what can be considered caring work is often bound up in the complex and enmeshed relationships between these individuals. Mr Sawyer, who was in his early 70s and caring for his wife of over 40 years, emphasized that he saw what he was doing as being related, not only to his long marriage, but also primarily to the love and concern he felt for his wife. For him this was not 'caring as such', but a desire to share with his wife:

> It can apply to a husband or wife who've been married for 40–50 years and are still in love with each other as much. So the word caring would probably not apply there. Be just love and concern for the other person. That's what the motivations would be. So that's my feeling about it.

In some families there was a precedent already in place for certain individual's to participate in such types of caregiving. This was true for both the daughters in the study, and was particularly strong in the case of Mrs Nash who was in her mid-40s and caring for her mother who lived a few streets away. She was married with two grown-up daughters and a teenage son. Mrs Nash was the only member of her mother's immediate family to be directly asked to look after her at home following her diagnosis:

> Well I used to work. Um, when Mum found out about her illness, um, she said would you be there at home with me in case I need you? And I said yes.

Neither of Mrs Nash's two brothers, who both lived locally, or her father had been asked to participate in caring for their mother. This did at times cause some resentment for Mrs Nash, particularly when she had to make fairly complicated arrangements for her own daughters to care for her mother when she went away for a few days. When Mrs Nash questioned her father about spending more time with his wife, he replied that he would do so only when the situation deteriorated further:

> And I have suggested to him why don't you cut down (working) and do a couple of days a week, you know. And he said 'If I feel that your mother is getting to the stage that she needs me to be there all the time I will.

Within this particular family there was also a very strong tradition of the daughters and women 'looking after' other family members. Mrs Nash's own mother had been involved in caring for her mother for 14 years until her death a few years previously, and it is possible that the implicit assumption within the family was that Mrs Nash, as the only daughter, would repeat the pattern her mother had set previously.

For Mrs Page, there had been a similar assumption of a traditional caring role being adopted, although for Mrs Page this was partly a consequence of both her brothers living a long distance away from her mother, whereas she lived in the next street. For Mrs Page the practical aspects of the caregiving role were shared towards the end of the study by the return home (to the same town) of one brother, which did relieve some of the burden of caring for their mother:

> I mean he has done quite well, and the other night when she called him in the night, well, half past eleven or whatever it was, um, she said to me on the Sunday 'You didn't mind?' 'No Mum,' I said, 'that's what we said, you know, let [brother] take a bit of the pressure

off', I said. After all [brother] didn't have to get up for work in the morning which I did, you know.

A further reason for the family caregivers participation in caregiving was a desire to return care given to them in the past by the ill person. Such caregiving reciprocity is one explanation for the provision of mutual aid and support within a relationship (Finch and Mason 1993), although it is not always clear how far such support should extend. For example the normative level of reciprocity between more extended family members, or individuals whose relationships have been changed by divorce or remarriage is unclear (Finch and Mason 1993). Mr Lloyd was the youngest family caregiver in the study at 37 years old, and was caring for his wife and their two young daughters and his step son, in addition to holding down a full-time job. For Mr Lloyd there was a definite sense of reciprocity in the caregiving he gave to his wife, although he accepted that the consequences of his wife's condition were somewhat different to the patterns of care she had extended to him in the past:

> 'Cos when you're actually married to someone you're there through thick and thin anyway aren't you? If I was ill she'd look after me, and if she was ill I'd look after her like, you know. Um, I remember when I was in hospital, I had two bad injuries playing rugby where I was put in hospital, and I had an operation. When I came out I couldn't, I was on crutches. Er, she always looked after me then. I mean it's just this is, I don't know, a bit longer that's all.

The family caregiver's story

The family caregiver's story was very embedded in the patient's story, and this was particularly true during the first interview. In subsequent interviews, although the patient's story still dominated much of the family caregiver's conversation, their own needs, concerns, and coping strategies began to emerge. The impact that the cared-for person's illness had on changing expectations and roles was extremely difficult for many family caregivers to identify. In some cases, where a couple had been married for many years, the enmeshed nature of their relationship made it even more difficult to distinguish between one spouse's story and the other. It is possible that in such relationships there was an implicit understanding and acceptance of each other's needs that was reflected in their joint story. However, it may also be that the accounts that individual family caregivers gave of the situation may be reflecting socially acceptable stories that privilege the ill person, particularly as this illness was known to be terminal. Furthermore, family caregivers may have felt that to concentrate on their own stories would be selfish, when the ill person clearly had a great need of understanding and care. Therefore, family caregivers' own stories and needs were often hidden and needed to be drawn out from the many implicit assumptions and expectations that were made about the caregiving situation.

Changing life roles and expectations

The progression of the cared-for persons illness often resulted in changes to the roles and expectations about the future held, either individually or jointly, by the family caregiver and the ill person. For the patient, one of the most significant life changes, for those under the age of retirement, was connected with work. The necessity of leaving employment or becoming long-term sick, or taking early retirement or redundancy, had financial as well as psychological consequences for the patient and also the family caregiver as they sought to support them during this time.

For the family caregivers' who were in employment, there were various degrees of support provided by their work that enabled them to undertake the caregiving role. Some employers were extremely sympathetic to the family caregiver's needs for time off work; for example, Mr Lloyd was given a different job that allowed him to work reduced hours, so that he could be available to look after his wife and children:

> They've [work] been really good to me since we found out. Um, I've had [a change of job] so I can get the time off to look after her. So job wise they've been really good to me.

Mrs Foster was in her mid-50s and was caring for her husband. Their two sons both lived over 60 miles away and were therefore unable to provide practical assistance. For this reason Mr and Mrs Foster appeared to rely on friends and neighbours, especially for assistance with transport to and from hospital appointments and maintaining their large garden.

Mrs Foster worked full time in a responsible position within a large office. She reported that her husband had found it quite difficult being at home all day when she was still at work full time:

> He's had to take early retirement . . . . Um, in fact he's talking about me not going to work full time any more because he'd like me to be around at home.

Whilst Mrs Foster wanted to support her husband and comply with his desire for her to be at home, she also enjoyed her work and felt that it gave her some 'time off' from thinking about the situation. This was the only form of escape she was able to control, and she was therefore reluctant to give this up.

For other family caregivers some employers were particularly unsympathetic towards the family caregiver's need for time off work, which was very upsetting at a time when anxiety and concern were already high. Mr Bradley, who was 61 years old, did not consider himself to be a carer but rather saw his role as part of his relationship responsibility towards his wife. They had been married for nearly 30 years and had no children. Mr Bradley had two sisters who lived some distance away (approximately 30 miles). In addition, Mrs Bradley had one sister who lived in Scotland but visited regularly, and one sister with whom they no longer had contact due to a family disagreement some years previously.

Mr Bradley had a close neighbour and friend who often came to visit his wife and sit with her so that he could go shopping. This neighbour had offered more help, but Mr Bradley did not want to make a habit of calling on her for assistance as she had her own family problems to deal with.

Mr Bradley had worked for his company for 38 years with very little sick leave and was hurt by the lack of compassion towards his circumstances and the particularly clumsy way that his case had been handled, for which his line manager later apologized. They had insisted that he take all his annual leave before his doctor signed him off sick to look after his wife:

I had to have me holidays, I took some of me holidays. But um, I thought there might have been some, you know, perhaps a little bit of compassion. I didn't expect to have months off, but the word profit the word profit was mentioned.

Not only did this increase his distress during his wife's final weeks, but had the potential to make things difficult for him on his return to work following his wife's death.

Another aspect, which was expressed by some of the younger family caregivers, was that plans and dreams about activities to be undertaken during retirement were clearly no longer going to be possible. Mrs White, a 49-year-old special needs teacher reported missing, and being angry about, the things that she would no longer be able to do with her husband:

Cheated . . . . Because of all the things that we were going to do. And we can't do. For [husband] more than myself I think. All the places that we looked round and . . . . Cheated on all the things that we can't do, or [husband] can't do, both of us really. Er, just go for a walk in the woods.

Mrs White was more concerned about her husband's loss of dreams and identity, which have been described as biographical disruption by Bury (1982), than her own. However, for the family caregivers who clearly shared a very enmeshed relationship with the ill person, such a threat to the shared dreams and expectations caused by the terminal diagnosis of cancer is likely to threaten their own sense of identity as well. By constantly placing the patient's needs over their own there was a tendency for the family caregiver to ignore or hide a recognition of their own forthcoming loss. This may well have enabled them to continue in the family caregiving role, but one consequence of this may be that they were less prepared for the death of their relative than would be anticipated in a palliative care setting, which stresses the importance of an open acknowledgement of the death of the ill person.

As a result of this openness regarding the prognosis of the ill person there was often a desire to accommodate the patient's desires and wishes as much as possible; for example, a desire to be cared for at home. The desire to fulfil the ill person's wishes was complied with even if the family caregiver did not believe this was necessarily in the cared-for person's best interests. Mr Bradley described how he would have preferred his wife to make more effort to get out while she still had the opportunity. His wife had been offered a place at the local hospice day centre, but only went approximately three times when she felt she wanted to, despite Mr Bradley feeling that is would be a good thing for her to do:

No I think I used to try to get her to go out somewhere, you know, like for a ride in the car and that. But, they have been trying recently tried to make sure she went to the hospice because it does give me that um, sort of four or five hours break . . . . But um, if she don't go well it's just one of those things, just carry on.

Although Mr Bradley believed that his wife would have had more pleasure on taking some trips out, he was content to allow her to choose how she spent her final few weeks, even though this resulted in him not being able to get a break from the caregiving role.

Coping strategies of the family caregiver

Family caregivers reported a number of strategies that they used to deal with the situation. Past experience of caring for other members of the family, with or without cancer, was a common feature in some of the stories. For some people their experience of cancer care was from a long time ago and they recognized that things would almost certainly be different now; for example, Mr Sawyer:

> Breast cancer it was you know. And um, I went through all they. Well the one of the one Aunt was very close to me she was my Godmother . . . . She'd seen what had happened to her sisters you see, and she took her own course. Because things were different then weren't they? We're talking about 40 years ago you know.

Many of the participants appeared to have a strong sense of identification with the patient, as observed in the way they talked about the patient and themselves in the same context, often using language such as 'we' and 'us' rather than 'I' and 'me'. For this reason it was sometimes hard to differentiate between the perspectives of the patient and the family caregiver. Some couples who had been married for a long time were often able to anticipate each other's sentences, and it may be that they did think about the situation in the same way as their identities had become so entwined over the years.

Learning to put a brave face on things so that the patient would not be upset was also common to many of the family caregivers. Mr Lloyd used laughter to help him deal with things, and reported finding the ribbing he received from his work mates as helpful in taking him out of himself for a period of time:

> I mean the lads in work, I mean they all take the Mick like, you know, but that's part of being in the job . . . . That probably does me good that does, going in. And even though I'm not there long like, just having the Mick taken out of me, and banter like that, perks me up when I'm feeling down.

Obtaining information about the situation, treatment, or prognosis was also a useful strategy for dealing with the situation, and was seen as important for both the patient and the family caregiver. When issues arose for the family caregivers that required professional information or expertise addressing these issues, either with health professionals involved in the situation or those who were not, enabled the family caregivers to deal more effectively with the situation. For example, Mrs Nash was particularly concerned about her mother's cancer and the implications this might have for her own health. As it proved difficult to talk to the visiting home care nurse without upsetting her mother, she decided to visit her own GP for information about the situation:

> I went and saw my own GP, when we, when they told us that Mum had this um, er, tumour on the ovary. I thought to myself well should I see my doctor and explain? . . . . And I said is there some sort of test that I should go through? And she said no, she said because it's very hard to detect and you can't always tell that its there until its too late, you know.

For Mrs Nash there was a lack of information surrounding her mother's cancer that had implications for her own health. By approaching her own GP, Mrs Nash was able to explore these issues with a health professional who was not attached to the situation and who could give her the information she required for her own health needs independently of her mother's care.

Family caregivers' liaison with health professionals

Family caregivers had a diversity of experience and familiarity with visiting health and social care professionals. Understanding the different roles of these health professionals was important for the family caregiver's ability to understand who and how to access different service providers. However, it was not clear how the family caregivers developed their knowledge of these different roles. It may be possible that their knowledge was built up over a period of time with increasing contact with health professionals. Thus, if a situation arose where professional input was required, the family caregiver would be able to identify the most appropriate person to contact. As most family caregivers visited during this study had been caring for some time, they appeared to have established to their own satisfaction who they would contact in different circumstances. Generally, there appeared to be a lack of any written literature available to family caregivers that differentiated between the roles of various health professionals. The knowledge of who was responsible for what aspects of the ill persons well-being therefore appeared to be learnt rather vicariously by many of the family caregivers. One family caregiver (Mrs White) did comment that she would have liked to have access to written information, particularly at the beginning of her husband's illness:

> At the very onset you are in such a whirl when you are told this is what is happening that you do need that information . . . . Go away and read this, you know, you're not going to feel like reading it but this is going to give you that help that you do need.

When health professionals were only seen periodically, for example, the occupational therapist (OT), there was less clear identification of role boundaries or accessibility to a service. Although Mrs Vaughan, with her long experience and involvement with the health care system, had no difficulty in identifying the professional boundaries between groups of health professionals:

> A district nurse actually just assesses people. 'Well I think you ought to have a doctor.' . . . . Macmillan nurse is more of a counsellor. A Macmillan nurse is not allowed to sit with a patient on her own, a Marie Curie Nurse does that . . . . They [Macmillan nurse] can't touch a person, they can look but they can't administer the drug . . . . [Hospice Doctor] he's a pain control doctor . . . . Well the occupational therapist is the person that assesses the patient to the equipment he requires in the home to lead what you call a good quality life.

Obviously there are a number of issues surrounding the boundaries between health professionals in this example. For example, the issue of what a Macmillan nurse is allowed to do and not do. Mrs Vaughan had a very clear idea that the Macmillan nurse did not fulfil the same role as the Marie Curie nurse.

Generally, family caregivers were more likely to seek information and advice from those health professionals with whom they had most contact. For example, Mr Bradley relied much more on the district nurses who were assisting him with the nursing care of his wife than the hospice nurse whom he only contacted if he required advice about some aspect of her treatment, particularly the drug regime:

> I mean [district nurses], they've all you know, what they've said I've gone along with. They are the people who are dealing with this sort of thing all the time aren't they? And you know you've got to take their advice.

Mrs Vaughan, on the other hand, was much more likely to contact the hospice nurse or the hospice itself if she had a query about her husband's condition, as she had much less contact with the district nurses:

> Because she's [hospice nurse] what you call my tie line between the hospice and home.

GPs and hospice doctors were generally only contacted after consultation with the visiting nurse, whether from the hospice or community, unless there was an emergency. This is not perhaps surprising as many of the family caregivers reported more contact with the nursing staff on a routine basis, even though some of the patients' GPs made an effort to keep in close contact, and in some situations would visit routinely. As more than one caregiver said, 'I don't want to waste their time, I know they're busy'. There is an implicit assumption that doctors are always busy and should therefore only be contacted or approached in an emergency. Some family caregivers used the hospice care nurses and district nurses as a means of accessing the doctors and legitimizing their need for a visit; for example, Mrs Vaughan:

> The district nurse is actually looking after the patient, she can actually assess the patient if he required any medical, she can refer that back to the doctor.

Not all family caregivers had experience of a particular service. In fact only a few mentioned having had contact with services outside of the hospice, community, or hospital teams. Those that had had previous contact with other services did feel able to contact them again, if there was a need, especially if there had been extensive use of a service. For example, Mrs Vaughan had contacted the OT when she felt her husband required more equipment in the home following his admission to the hospice.

During the course of the study it became increasingly clear that some individual family caregivers were referred to social care staff, such as that provided by social services. In particular, home care and social workers were involved with several of the family caregivers. Social care was provided for five of the sixteen family caregivers. Two younger (under 60 years of age) family caregivers and three older family caregivers were in receipt of social care, which consisted of assistance with personal care such as bathing for the ill person and some household chores and preparation of meals. For the older family caregivers, the provision of social care had been initiated prior to the diagnosis of cancer. For the younger family caregivers, provision of social care was requested when it became clear that the ill person's condition had deteriorated and the family caregiver could no longer manage to provide all the care required alone. For example, the visiting hospice nurse suggested that Mrs White might benefit from additional help when her husband's condition deteriorated. Mrs White requested that someone might help with the household chores in order for her to be able to concentrate on giving more personal care to her husband:

> That was organized because when [husband] was very bad, just before then it was suggested that we needed some form of home help . . . . They do the hoovering, er they hoover through and she washes the kitchen floor and bathroom floor, and the downstairs loo.

This does not mean that the remaining caregivers were not in need of more practical help, but that they had not been referred into the social care system at the time of the study. It is unclear what effect the changing patterns of social care in the community will have on the future support of this group of family caregivers.

Availability and approachability of health professionals

The level of perceived support available to the family caregivers from health professionals is an important aspect of the caregiving situation. Some family caregivers appeared only to want to know that health professionals were available to talk to if necessary and would rarely, if ever, contact them. These family caregivers would often be prepared to wait until the health professional contacted them, either by regular appointments or telephone contact, although they could always ask her/him to call earlier if necessary.

However, for Mrs Nash, access to the visiting health professional was blocked by her mother. This appeared to be primarily because she was concerned that issues would be discussed about her illness and treatment that were being kept from her:

> You see if I try to speak to [hospice nurse] then my Mum feels that I'm talking behind her back. I mean I've only got to see [hospice nurse] out the door and if I'm not straight back she'll say what are you talking about? Are you talking about me?

In fact Mrs Nash was particularly concerned about the implications for her own health following her mother's diagnosis, and eventually sought reassurance and information from her own GP.

Generally most communication with health professionals was concerned with the welfare and care of the patient, and there was little or no opportunity to discuss the family caregiver's own reactions to the situation or concerns for their own well-being. This may well be the result of the family caregiver's focus on putting the patient first (often because of a perceived limited time-span) or perhaps due to a misconception of the role of the health professional in relation to their own well-being.

Enquiries about the family caregiver's concerns or feelings appeared to focus on general polite questions regarding how they were coping with the situation, often at the end of a visit. Few of the family caregivers talked about the health professionals as a means of emotional support in the situation, although they clearly found their presence and the expertise that they brought to the situation helpful.

Health professionals were generally only referred to for information and advice about the medication and treatment of the patient and possible side-effects experienced, rather than supportive emotional care. Perhaps it is just this informational advice that is indeed the most helpful thing health professionals can contribute to the situation. That is, they can almost certainly provide guidelines for the family caregiver about expectations of treatment regimes and symptom control. This reassurance may be all that the family caregiver and the patient expect from health professionals. If this is the case, it is interesting to ask why this might be. Is it perhaps due to the pervasive notion of the ideal of family caregiving (Keating *et al.* 1994; Clark 1995), and the responsibility and obligation of family members to provide care for their relatives (Finch and Mason 1993; Finch 1995)? Or could this be due to the implicit assumption that family caregivers are acting from a desire to return care given in the past, or presumed to be available in the future, which results in an altruistic attitude focusing on the individual requiring care? If the reasons for giving care are reciprocity and altruistic behaviour, there would be little expectation by family caregivers of receiving emotional support from health professionals. Rather they would require specific and focused information and advice about how to carry out their caregiving role. Emotional support would therefore be expected to come from another source, although it is questionable if support can be allocated in this mechanistic way.

The emergence of the family caregiver role

Many of the family caregivers acted, often unconsciously, as a legitimate source of information about the ill person's status for the health professionals. In this respect, family caregivers could be thought of as a co-ordinator between the visiting health and social care professionals, both at home and from the hospital or hospice settings. For example, as family caregivers were almost always involved in consultations between the ill person and health professionals throughout the illness trajectory, they held a great deal of information about the ill person's progress, suggested treatments, and changes in the ill person's care. Furthermore, some of the cared-for people requested that the family caregiver be present whenever there was a consultation with medical personnel, as they were not always able to understand or take on board the implications and changes proposed in treatments. Thus, some family caregivers had more accurate information about the situation than the ill person themselves. For example, Mr Lloyd:

> Well [wife] don't take a lot of it in while she's in there anyway see. And this is one of the reasons why she says to me you have to come along because its not sinking in me head.

By taking on responsibility and acting as an advocate for the ill person during medical and nursing consultations, the family caregiver often became very proficient at communicating with other health professionals who may need to know and understand the latest suggestions for treatment. For example, the most common topic of conversation with the health professional was reported to be concerning the patient and their current symptoms and status.

Within this co-ordinating role, the family caregiver also developed certain expertise about dealing with the situation. This involved understanding the treatment regime itself, which could be quite involved; for example, Mrs Foster:

> They decided that they would do this stem cell replacement treatment . . . . [He] went in for a week's intensive chemo, and came home and had hormone injections which boosts apparently the cells out of the bone marrow and into the blood and that was harvested . . . . Then they did the stem cell replacement which the weeks chemo knocked out all your immune system completely, and the stem cell was obviously supposed to

boost it back up. He was quite ill several times, but we got through that and we came home . . . . They did a scan and said well it had gone, its shrunk from about the size of a grapefruit to about the size of a walnut, but its not gone.

And also general nursing care of the ill person; for example, Mr Bradley:

I mean they tell me about her medication and what, you know, what to do, how to go about things and that.

For the family caregiver prioritising issues surrounding the ill person's care with the health professional could result in a decreased opportunity to discuss more personal and emotional issues relating to the situation.

Implications for professional practice

This chapter has begun to explore the perception of a group of family caregivers in relation to the role of 'carer' in palliative care and the nature of the relationship with visiting health professionals. It became clear that there was a degree of ambiguity for family caregivers regarding identification with the term 'carer'. This ambiguity became a predominant focus of the interaction between family caregivers and health professionals, as both sought to define and negotiate the role of 'carer' within palliative care. For those family caregivers who had been involved in the health care system for some time, there appeared to have developed an implicit understanding of what was expected of them as a carer. However, for those individuals who did not identify with the term carer, there appeared to be inconsistencies in the nature of their relationship with health professionals. For example, they were often unable to access support for their own emotional and physical needs from health professionals, except when those needs impinge on the patient's requirements or wishes. The lack of clear understanding of the term carer could also be a source of possible confusion and misunderstanding about expectations and limitations of an individual's ability to perform the role of carer in this situation.

To avoid confusion as to the role and activities a family caregiver may be able and willing to undertake, it is important to recognize any differences in the perception of the term 'carer' between health professionals and individual family caregivers. By more clearly defining the role of carer within palliative care, there will be less likelihood of family members being unexpectedly placed in the position of accepting a role or level of responsibility with which they may feel uncomfortable. In addition, openly acknowledging the family caregiver's rights and needs within the plan of care for the ill person may help to reduce the ambiguous position of this role. If the term carer is to be used to apply to family caregivers, it should be clearly stated and explicitly defined; limitations relating to the role and expectations of the individual will then be less contentious.

Gaining an insight into the perception that family caregivers hold of their place in palliative care can help the health professional to understand some of the implications of adopting this role. Furthermore, detailed understanding of the effect that caring has on the life of the family caregiver can also help the health professional to give more specific support to both the ill person and the family caregiver who is supporting them.

Summary

This chapter has explored the findings of a small-scale longitudinal study exploring the perception and support of family caregivers of someone with a terminal cancer diagnosis. Case study research was used to illustrate the themes across time for individual family members. Family caregivers' identification with the role of carer and their relationship with visiting health professionals were discussed. It was concluded that not all family caregivers identify with the term carer, and often saw their role as more closely related to kinship and familial responsibilities. In addition, family caregivers had a diversity of experience and familiarity with visiting health and social care professionals, which influenced their interactions with this group. Finally, some implications for health professional practice were considered.

References

Addington-Hall, J. and McCarthy, M. (1995). Dying from cancer: results of a national population-based investigation. *Palliative Medicine*, 9, 295–305.

Addington-Hall, J., MacDonald, L., Anderson, H., and Freeling, P. (1991). Dying from cancer: the views of bereaved family and friends about the experiences of terminally ill patients. *Palliative Medicine*, 5, 207–214.

Arber, S. and Gilbert, N. (1989). Men: the forgotten carers. *Sociology*, 23, 111–118.

Arber, S. and Ginn, J. (1990). The meaning of informal care: gender and the contribution of Elderly people. *Aging and Society*, 10, 429–454.

Bury, M. (1982). Chronic illness as biographical disruption. *Sociology of Health and Illness*, 4, (2), 167–182.

Carey, P. J., Oberst, M. T., McCubbin, M. A., and Hughes, S. H. (1991). Appraisal and caregiving burden in family members caring for patients receiving chemotherapy. *Oncology Nursing Forum*, 8, (8), 1341–1348.

Clark, L. (1995). Family care and changing family structure: bad news for the elderly? In *The future of family care for older people* (ed. I. Allen and E. Perkins), p. 19–49. HMSO, London.

Duke, S. (1998). An exploration of anticipatory grief: the lived experience of people during their spouses' terminal illness and in bereavement. *Journal of Advanced Nursing*, 28, (4), 829–839.

Field, D. (1995). *Special not different: GP's accounts of terminal care.* Paper delivered to the British Sociological Association Annual Conference, Leicester, July 1995.

Finch, J. (1995). Responsibilities, obligations and commitments. In *The future of family care for older people* (ed. I. Allen and E. Perkins), p. 51–64. HMSO, London.

Finch, J. and Mason, J. (1993). *Negotiating family responsibilities.* Routledge, London.

Heaton, J. (1999). The gauze and visibility of the carer: a Foucauldian analysis of the discourse of informal care. *Sociology of Health and Illness*, 21, (6), 759–777.

Hinton, J. (1994). Can home care maintain an acceptable quality of life for patients with terminal cancer and their relatives? *Palliative Medicine*, 8, 183–196

Keating, N., Kerr, K., Warren, S., Grace, M., and Wertenberger, D. (1994). Who's the family in family caregiving? *Canadian Journal on Aging*, 13, (2), 268–287.

Neale, B. and Clark D. (1992). Informal palliative care. *Journal of Cancer Care*, 3, 85–89.

Nekolaichuk, C. L., Maguire, T. O., Suarez-Almazor, M., Rogers W. T., and Bruera, E. (1999). Assessing the reliability of patient, nurse, and family caregiver symptom ratings in hospitalized advanced cancer patients. *Journal of Clinical Oncology*, **17**, (11), 3621–3630

Neufeld, A. and Harrison, M.J. (1998). Men as caregivers: reciprocal relationships or obligation? *Journal of Advanced Nursing*, **28**, (5), 959–968.

Nolan, M., Keady J., and Grant, G. (1995). Developing a typology of family care: implications for nurses and other service providers. *Journal of Advanced Nursing*, **21**, 256–265

Nolan, M., Grant, G., and Keady, J. (1996). *Understanding family care: a multidimensional model of caring and coping*. Open University Press, Buckingham.

Pitkeathley, J. (1989). *It's my duty isn't it? The plight of carers in our society*. Souvenir Press, London.

Rose, K.E. (1998). Perceptions related to time in a qualitative study of informal carers of terminally ill cancer patients. *Journal of Clinical Nursing*, **7**, 343–350.

Rose, K.E. (1999). A qualitative analysis of the information needs of informal carers of terminally ill cancer patients. *Journal of Clinical Nursing*, **8**, 81–88.

Seale, C. (1989). What happens in hospices: A review of research evidence. *Social Science Medicine*, **28**, (6), 551–559.

Seale, C. and Cartwright, A. (1994). *The year before death*. Aldershot, Avebury.

Spackman, A. (1991). The health of informal carers. *Institute for Health Policy Studies*. University of Southampton, Southampton.

The Carers National Association. (1996). *Facts about carers*. Ruth Pitter House, London.

Theis, S. and Deitrick, E. (1987). Respite care: a community needs survey. *Journal of Community Health Nursing*, **4**, 85–92.

Thorpe, G. (1993). Enabling more dying to remain at home. *British Medical Journal*, **307**, 915–918.

Twigg, J. (1989). Models of carers: how do social care agencies conceptualise their relationship with informal carers? *Journal of Social Policy*, **18**, (1), 53–66.

Twigg, J., Atkin, K., and Perring, C. (1990). *Carers and services: a review of research*. Social Policy Research Unit (SPRU), HMSO.

Yin, R.B. (1994). *Case study research: design and methods*, (2nd edn). Sage Publications, London.

Chapter 6

Being a carer in acute crisis: the situation for relatives of organ donors

Magi Sque

Introduction

Many chronic illnesses have stages of acute crisis that, at times, may terminate in unexpected, sudden death. Most studies to date appear to focus on provision for specific needs rather than on an attempt to describe 'the life-world' of the family and what it is actually like to be a relative of a loved one who is dying or newly dead. Costain-Schou and Hewison (1999) voiced their concern at the lack of social insight provided by previous measurement studies about carers and the cared for. In failing to investigate the social context, an informative picture cannot be adequately developed of the quality of life of carers, of what it consists, and how it is to be maximized and safeguarded. Therefore a shift is needed toward approaches that better capture the complexity and uniqueness, and focus on the role of personal meanings, to achieve an understanding of how families view their situation and cope with their often profoundly poignant and rueful circumstances.

This chapter draws on the experiences of being a carer confronted with acute critical injury, experiences that could illuminate other life-threatening or end-of-life situations. The themes discussed are taken from a narrative interview study of the experiences of 24 relatives of multi-organ donors. The study sought to elicit an understanding of the nature and meaning of having a relative in a critical care situation that ended in organ donation. A theory of 'dissonant loss' was developed to explain this type of bereavement and explicate the needs of relatives (Sque 1996; Sque and Payne 1996). Grounded theory (Glaser and Strauss 1967) was used to develop an understanding of relatives' experiences of organ donation. This approach facilitated a model of client care based on the actual experiences of the individuals involved, rather than a prescriptive approach of what problems are thought to be important or relevant by professionals who may not have direct experience of the phenomena themselves.

The theory of dissonant loss not only provides for the special case of relatives of organ donors but also speaks to the experiences of carers caught in acute, critical crisis and issues that this manifests for them. The next section will describe the theory of dissonant loss and will be followed by sections on: An environment for conflict—relatives reactions to critical injury and hospitalization; Conflict and resolution in the confirmation of brainstem death, in donation decisions, and in saying goodbye; 'What do I do now?'; and Conflict and resolution in the bereavement process.

The theory of dissonant loss

Letters facilitated by transplant co-ordinators from three Regional Transplant Co-ordinating Services in England invited a purposive sample of relatives from 42 families to join the study. Relatives were chosen for their perceived wide range of experiences of organ donation, such as their relationship to the donor and geographical location, which could have affected availability of bereavement support. Sixteen families (24 relatives) agreed to join the study, six families declined, three were overseas, and 17 did not reply. Participating relatives consisted of husbands, wives and parents, and a daughter-in-law. Audio-taped, narrative interviews were carried out in their homes. Twelve donations were requested and four were offered spontaneously.

Analyses of interview transcripts were guided by a grounded theory approach, based on the constant comparative method. The in-depth interviews examined participants' emotional reactions to the critical injury, death, and donation, perceptions of the decision-making process, and assessment of the problems donation had caused for them, as well as the benefits it provided. These topics were used to inform the analyses. By the end of data collection, a clustering of concepts were classified into themes that were used to form 11 definitive categories. The categories were arranged around the central purpose of the research, *donor relatives' experiences*, to form an analytical version of their story. The model in Fig. 6.1 shows the conceptual representation of this story.

The model indicates a sequential relationship of these categories that described participants commonly constructed realities of the donation experience. These were: 'The last time we were together,' Finding out something is wrong, Waiting for a diagnosis, Hopes and expectations, Becoming aware things are going wrong, Realization of death, Confirmation of brainstem death, Donation decisions, Saying goodbye, 'What do I do now?' and Dealing with grief and donation.

There appeared to be particular behaviours through which participants acted out each phase. These were:

- recalling—when participants talked about the attributes of their relative and the last occasion they shared together;
- informing—when they were first told something had gone wrong;
- hoping—during the hospital experience;
- realizing—that their relative would not recover;
- deciding—about donation;
- parting—leaving the relative;
- coping—with grief and donation.

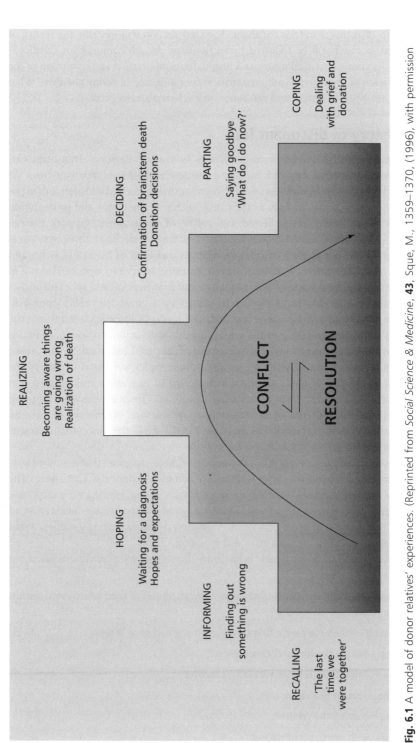

Fig. 6.1 A model of donor relatives' experiences. (Reprinted from *Social Science & Medicine*, **43**, Sque, M., 1359–1370, (1996), with permission from Elsevier Science.)

Sque, M., and Payne, S. (1996) Dissonant Loss: the experiences of donor relatives Social Science and Medicine 43, (9), 1359–1370. [Copyright year 1996] For Figs: 6.1, 6.2

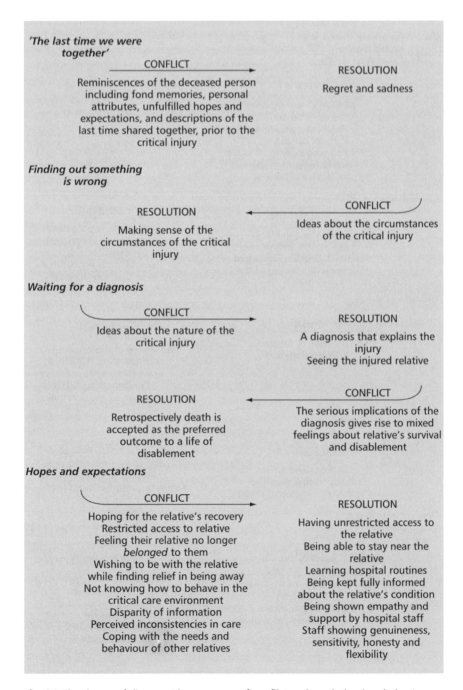

Fig. 6.2 The theory of dissonant loss: sources of conflict and resolution in relatives' experience of critical illness and organ donation. (Reprinted from *Social Science & Medicine*, **43**, Sque, M., 1359–1370, (1996), with permission from Elsevier Science.)

Becoming aware things are going wrong
Realization of death

CONFLICT

Knowing recovery is no
longer possible
Personal realization
of death
Not knowing how to behave
Waiting for confirmation
of brainstem death

RESOLUTION

Confirmation of
brainstem death

Confirmation of BSD

RESOLUTION

Confidence in BSDT
Not seeing the relative once
brainstem death is confirmed
Post retrieval viewing of the
body

CONFLICT

Difficult to equate death
with the appearance of
the ventilated relative
Lack of knowledge about
brainstem death testing

Donation Decisions

CONFLICT

Decisions to be made
about donation

RESOLUTION

Knowledge of the donor's wishes
Attributes of the donor
Personal realisation of death
Confirmation of BSD
Information about retrieval

Saying Goodbye
'What do I do now?'

RESOLUTION

Options and advice
about 'saying goodbye'
Post retrieval telephone call

CONFLICT

Leaving a person who does
not appear to be dead
Aesthetic presentation of the body

Dealing with grief
and donation

CONFLICT

Termination of the affectional
bonds for parts of the relative
that live on
Donation decisions
Lack of bereavement support

RESOLUTION

Focusing on the achievement
of the donor
Information about the
recipients
Feeling of making a
contribution
Knowing some good has
come out of the death
The donation is recognised,
valued and not forgotten
Specialist bereavement
support

BSDT=Brainstem death test
BSD =Brainstem death

These behaviours were explained through a process of conflict and resolution, which pervaded the categories and formed the core variable of participants' experience. Conflict is defined in this sense as:

> The simultaneously opposing tendencies within the individual or environment, which cause discrepancy, discord, or dissonance, and the distress resulting from these instances.

The study describes factors that created resolutions to participants' conflicts and helped them move through the phases of donation process. Using the core variable a theory of 'dissonant loss' was developed to explain participants' concerns during the donation experience, shown in Fig. 6.2.

Dissonant loss is defined as:

> A bereavement or loss, which is characterized by a sense of uncertainty and psychological inconsistency.

The loss is assured but the effects of the loss are surrounded by ambiguity and incompatibility with the participants' assumptive world (Parkes 1971, 1993). Dissonance occurs as the loss involves a series of complex decisions made necessary by the ubiquitous and pervasive elements of conflict and resolution. Conflict originated in the short and intensely emotional period of hospitalization. During this time participants appeared to lose control to the professionals, as they were functioning outside of their familiar world.

The degree of conflict and dissonance experienced by participants was compounded by a lack of experience and knowledge about the events of organ donation and retrieval. It was within this environment that participants were asked to make complex decisions about donation that had implications for their own emotional well-being and ability to manage their bereavement.

Within the context of bereavement, donor relatives like other carers faced with a tragic and sudden death (of a relatively young person, who for all intents and purposes was previously healthy or stable in their disease process) are at high risk of aberrant bereavement outcomes (Yates *et al.* 1990; Wright 1996; Sque 2000). The unexpected nature of the death may make its acceptance difficult for families to reconcile. Next-of-kin are necessarily approached about organ donation when their grief may be all-encompassing, and thinking and concentration a problem. However, if donation is to take place, families need to make a number of decisions on behalf of their deceased relative. These decisions may be problematic, as they concern an operation on another's body; yet, the time to debate the issues is limited. Relatives are asked to accept a non-stereotypical death, brainstem death, as death. The implications of brainstem death transcend the usual experience of the lay individual. The potential donor maintained on a ventilator may not look dead, and often has no external manifestations of injury; they tend to be unscathed, resting, warm, florid, and their chest moves as if they are breathing; they may even move occasionally if a spinal reflex is activated. Their time of death becomes an arbitrary decision made by the attending physicians. Not only are relatives asked to accept this situation as death, but also they are asked to agree to the removal of the very vital organs that normally would maintain life.

Sque and Payne's (1996) work suggested that the experience of organ donation could be explained as bereavement characterized by a series of complex decisions, accompanied by a sense of uncertainty and psychological inconsistency. Similar situations in acute illness crisis may produce the need for carers to make complex decisions about continuing or terminating life-sustaining interventions, and may encompass issues that surround what is perceived and desired in a dignified death, and the care and disposal of the body.

An environment for conflict—relatives' reactions to critical injury and hospitalization

Information that the relative had sustained an injury was reported to the participants in a variety of ways. Nine families were informed via the telephone, which was described by a participant, as leaving a lasting memory. Four were present when the relative collapsed. Two were informed by friends or other relatives, who themselves had telephone calls and went in search of the participants. One participant received information about his daughter's accident from the police, who came to his house. These first communications were often scant. Witnessing a collapse at home for participants was a bewildering and frightening experience, because the nature of these events was unexpected, sudden, and primarily unexplained. The following extract describes a mother's experience with her baby and her reactions:

> I saw that he was yellow and I couldn't understand why he was so cold. It was only when I went over to him I saw a trickle of blood coming down his mouth. Well I just can't explain what went through me then . . . calling out for my next door neighbour. I called out to her twice, so she came over and I said, 'My baby is dead,' . . . she held him and that was it then, I just had to get away from him, I just felt so frightened, I just didn't want to see him, just really, really frightened.

Relatives who became sick at home were transferred to hospital by ambulance. In some cases participants travelled in the ambulance, as once there was recognition that the relative was seriously ill there appeared to be a desire to remain close to them. This reaction to wish to remain close to the loved one is a consistent theme across much research into caring, Pelletier's (1993a) work with donor families described the importance of 'keeping the connection' while Walters (1995) stated that the emotional and physical presence of 'being with and seeing the patient' was helpful to families. A mother reported the great comfort she experienced over the intervening months after the death of her son, in that, while travelling in the ambulance with him he shouted out, 'Mum', and that was the last word he spoke, and she felt he knew she was there.

It was during the initial encounters with hospital personnel that relatives got the first clues to the extent of the injury and the diagnosis and prognosis of the patient, as generally they arrived at the hospital with very little information:

> I would say at this point we didn't know then how gravely injured M had been.

Participants had an early need to try and make sense of what had happened so suddenly to their relative. They needed to, 'Try and build up a picture of what happened':

> There was speculation that there was tractors going up and down the very narrow road or it could have been a bee, could have been the horse she had trailing her you know, on

a lead, could have bit the other one, could have been anything that made the horse rear, there is no conclusive evidence to say what it was, the tractor driver that was approaching he . . . he witnessed her falling off.

Some participants tended to draw parallels with past experience to help them make sense of what was happening. This could be helpful or create further anxiety for them when past experiences had ended in poor outcomes. Others found the circumstance of the injury unacceptable and blamed certain things or people for causing or contributing to its effect.

Seeing the relative for the first time and hearing the medical opinion of the illness were the two major features of this part of participants' experience. There was a need for participants to know the diagnosis and the trajectory of the relative's injury to help them make sense of what was happening. What was most important to participants was that they were kept fully informed about anything that affected their relative. Participants appreciated being told what was being done and what would happen next, such as the relative being moved to the Intensive Care Unit (ICU), and being prepared, by the nurses, for seeing them. Participants sometimes had to take the initiative to get information about the relative. Sykes *et al.* (1992) stated that relatives needed to be kept updated about the changes in the condition of the patient with regard to prognosis and progress, and that carers' experiences at time of death could often colour their assessment of all the services received during the patients' terminal illness. They described the difficulty of trying to take in information in their state of shock:

> You try so hard to listen so you don't miss anything that you don't take it in, it just goes above your head, none of us could remember you know what they said.

Diagnosis was also important in informing participants, where appropriate, that they had acted in the best possible manner to try to save the life of their relative. Where effort was put into securing a diagnosis, families were very appreciative. On occasion doctors would show participants the results of scans; this did help them to understand the extent of the injury:

> Anyway, the doctor came along and said would you like to have a look at the scan thing for yourself and we went over and had a look and I could see how massive it was. I never seen anything as big as that thing because I'd seen scans myself in my work and I thought wow!

However, participants reported their acute distress at learning the diagnosis, as well as, 'Mixed feelings', when they knew that if the relative lived they would have been severely disabled. This notion of 'disablement' also appears to be used as a coping strategy when death was confirmed, as it was thought that such a life would not have been acceptable to the individual:

> All those things flash through your mind and you always come into conflict with what you are thinking, don't you, shouldn't be thinking like this, should we think like that, should we do this, should we do that, really it's a funny thing to be sitting through because it's all so unreal isn't it, because every thought you have you have to contradict yourself and yeah, but I am sure what happened was for the best in regards to that, because being brain damaged and not having a life at all, from the one she wanted, lets put it that way.

Participants found waiting difficult. Time spent away from the relative was particularly difficult. Participants were torn between the need to be close to their loved one, 'I couldn't bear to be away from her, I had to be with her', and the benefit they thought the relative was getting from highly technical, medical interventions. A mother wary of upsetting any of her son's monitoring equipment reports how given access and encouragement she gained confidence in approaching her baby son and was able to renew the bonding process:

> I sort of slept by his feet and I was always holding him, because when he first went into hospital even though I felt better for seeing him breathing and the proper colour and everything I just could not touch him, and the following days I was able to hold his hand, and then I sort of tried to cuddle him and then I kissed him and then I felt more comfortable, even though he was my own baby I was very petrified at the beginning . . . then the hours ticked, I felt the bond, there was always been a bond . . .

Participants' uncomfortable feelings, coupled with the nature of the interventions and the need to make sense of what was happening, were found to create a special need for communication that kept them fully informed about the patient's condition.

It was important to participants to feel that the health care professionals cared about the patient and that this was demonstrated in their technical and personal involvement, and in their actions, words, and presence, 'being there.' To know that everything humanly and medically possibly was being done for the patient had been noted to be important to families. A participant, although she was satisfied with, 'The really good care' her relative got, thought that the nurses, 'Laughing and mucking about in the office', just seemed, 'unkind', when the family was in such a state of distress. The most appreciated qualities in staff were genuineness, sensitivity, honesty, and flexibility. A husband reports his feelings about the Sister in charge:

> Because she sort of took us under her wing and sort of looked after us like a mother hen, she really was, she came over, very, I suppose, from an emotional point of view she had empathy for us and was very, very supportive and she could care we were upset, she didn't show she was upset at all but what she did show was that she cared, she cared for us and if there was anything she could do better for us.'

However, another husband felt that senior staff were largely insensitive. He describes them as, 'Prima donnas in high tech medicine'. He felt his wife was, 'Treated as an abstract entity', being performed upon.

Relatives generally played little part in physical care. They were not encouraged to be involved by the nurses. They felt:

> I don't think there is a lot we could have done because there were so many wires and such like, no, I don't think, no, there was not a lot we could have done, being honest.

Participants felt this might have been different if the patient was conscious:

> I suppose had he been sort of conscious, yeah, we would probably have done something but because he was in a coma, whatever, it was better for them to, because they knew what they were doing, we would have, we might have done more harm than good.'

However, there were things that relatives did manage to get involved in as they commented that:

> Time does drag because you are there and after a while you feel inadequate, you're actually doing nothing but you are emotionally drained.

> It was hard feeling so inadequate and useless.

A young mother was encouraged to express milk to feed her baby during his hospitalization and was able to dress him at the end.

> I dressed him, put his nappy and everything on even though he had disposables because I always [used] Terries [type of nappy] on him, I dressed him as best as I could, wiped his face and everything.

Another participant accompanied his wife to the operating theatres and some did mouth care. Participants were also encouraged to talk to the relative as they were told that hearing is the last sense to be lost in coma. On one occasion, however, when a wife brought in a tape for her husband to listen to, 'The nurse took it away and said, 'he doesn't need that', but it made the wife feel better as she felt that she had done something to help. Participants found having a one-way conversation without privacy and with nurses they hardly knew present, awkward and difficult at first. However, over time they felt that the nurses made it easier, as they talked so naturally to the relative, which helped them to do likewise. They mainly spent time sitting by the bed, speaking to the relative, holding or touching and sometimes reading to them.

Participants constantly watched over the relative and were sometimes the first to notice that things were going wrong with the relative:

> Just knew that there was something going on, knew he wasn't, I knew he was sort of fading because he had this catheter bag at the side of the bed and it just kept filling up, pumping out water, it was like water all the time and I thought 'That isn't a very good sign anyway'. Then I thought, he was shooting it out, and then I kept saying [to the nurse] you're going to have to change this it is filling up, you will have to do something.

And they privately played a monitoring role:

> All we did was kept an eye on that monitor.

A father was able to maintain some control over access to his daughter by visitors who seemingly wanted, 'To gloat'. He felt she, 'Was not a show', and did seem to find some comfort through this stance in coping with his situation. He, 'Felt in control'. The importance of this control could be that he felt he was acting on behalf of his daughter and managing things the way she would have wanted, i.e. protecting her as he always had done, and getting her the best care and attention by not allowing her to become an object of curiosity. However, in many ways participants felt powerless:

> I think a lot of it is when you have somebody who is your family, they're close to you, but when they go into one of these places like this, they don't feel as if they are yours any more. You know, you feel as if you are just looking on. Somebody else or they have taken over, they're in the best care obviously . . . but you just feel as if you're perhaps outside looking in, as if they are nothing to do with you.

Significant others often had to provide explanations and comfort to other relatives and cope with family members' reactions that were sometimes seen as an added burden:

> And then my in-laws arrived, who I really don't get on with very well, and they caused a bit of a scene, they couldn't sit down and they were saying about the traffic was bad, and I just wanted them to shut up.

Others were sometimes concerned about the way that family members behaved. One father and mother were concerned about the, 'Embracive [*sic*] attitude', of two aunts, who were judged to speak, 'Indiscriminately', and, 'Wanted everything doing'. They were seen, 'To give the nurses a hard time', and the father eventually had to tell the nurses, 'Don't listen to them, he's my son'.

In other situations, as with participants in this study, carers may also have to cope with feelings of powerlessness, separatedness, isolation, and even fear, that can stem from barriers to physical contact with their loved ones. All carers are rarely without other obligations and responsibilities. It seemed to be a desire of study participants to retain a sense of 'normality' at home and a genuine desire that activities that affected the routine of children and animals should be maintained uninterrupted. These home commitments were often limiting factors on the time that participants could spend in hospital, and in some ways did help them to retain a sense of the 'real world' as they had other things outside the hospital to arrange and think about.

Whether in hospital, hospice, or home, studies have reported the need for carers to escape periodically from their caring roles. Where physical avoidance is not possible, relatives have been known to use alcohol, psychotropic medication, work, exercise, or simply refusing to believe their predicament (Pelletier 1993a). Lawton (2000) wrote that often relatives who could not escape their caring duties became closely enmeshed with the patient's own identity and sense of self, particularly when the patient's deterioration and level of dependency was very extreme. In taking over the functions and actions of another person's dependent body, carers experienced a fundamental change in their own sense of self. The patient's dependent body came to dictate their lifestyle and selfhood. In support of this argument Lawton (2000) states that comments frequently recounted by carers were:

> I felt so trapped.

> I've been leading someone else's [life] my mother's I suppose.

> I feel as if I have become mother to my mother.

In this study and others (Franz *et al.* 1997), participants spoke of, 'A desperate hope of a miracle'. Hope is a powerful motivator. It is the strongest theme in family studies and its importance is consistent across a number of studies, starting with Molter's (1979) seminal work, where relatives were asked to grade the items of care most important to them, through to Burnhill's (1999) exploration of anticipatory grief in an Italian population. In Burnhill's (1999) study, relatives identified the time from terminal diagnosis to death as a 'Journey of Hope'. Their experience was seen as a pilgrimage—Calvary, but where hope, although it changed its focus, was always present. Whether hope for a miracle, hope in the treatment, and hope of a cure—

through to hope of a comfortable and pain-free death for the relative. And I would suggest that for this study population hope, even after death, of improving a tissue or organ recipient's life. Molter (1979) and Burnhill (1999) and others suggest that hope acts to comfort relatives, sustains family support and relationships, and should never be denied.

Conflict and resolution in the confirmation of brainstem death

The time between the social acceptance of death and the objective confirmation of clinical death was shown to be especially difficult for participants, as they privately questioned their convictions of death occurring, and experienced difficulties in coping with the enquiries of friends and family, while feeling uncomfortable in continuing a relationship with what some perceived to be a ventilated corpse. These events lead some participants to desire an early end to the perceived suffering of their relative and the family with the confirmation of death:

> I couldn't see A lying in the bed in that condition being artificially kept alive, although I no longer, I no longer believed he was alive, I just believed that his body was functioning and so, I wanted to see him released from that and I wanted to see him prove one way or the other, with the least discomfort to him, and so they started to reduce the sedatives and at the end of that time they carried out, and I asked to be at the brainstem test at that stage.

> P said he'd like to bring the last brainstem forward because he could see what it was doing to me, and I agreed.

It was shown that relatives experienced considerable conflict in accepting brainstem death as death, due to the viable, unscathed physical appearance of the deceased; a finding supported by Savaria *et al.* (1990), Johnson (1992), Field (1993), Pelletier (1993a), and Douglass and Daly (1995). Plus, the ventilated maintenance of body function may have emphasized their similarity to other critically ill but clearly living patients. Here a father explains this difficulty for his family after he attended the brainstem-death testing of his son:

> It's an absolute shock to see conclusively that a person is no longer alive, that, that, they are dead. Then they put the respirator tube back into A's mouth and we went out. I had to go down and tell them (rest of the family) that I am afraid there was no hope now, that A was dead and that I saw no point in us remaining in the hospital at that stage but we should go and say goodbye to A, who was still looking comfortable rosy and warm, looking very much as if he was still alive. So it was very difficult for the other members of the family to understand that he was dead but I knew beyond any doubt that he was.

Participants found a number of ways to deal with the complex issue of time of death. For instance, some decided not to see the ventilated relative once brainstem death was confirmed. Others had confidence in the outcome of brainstem-death tests that appeared to be coupled with their own sense of death already occurring. Others were reassured by visiting with the body post-retrieval. Relatives need unambiguous information about the time of death, as alterations and misinformation were shown to cause distress. They are denied a moment of death that in Western culture assumes a sacred and revered quality (Fulton *et al.* 1987); an issue supported in studies by Coupe (1991), Soukup (1991), and Tymstra *et al.* (1992). Borozny (1988), Shanteau and Linin (1990), and Jasper *et al.* (1991) have pointed out that the decision to donate could be affected if brainstem death is regarded as less than permanent.

Conflict was exacerbated by the lack of knowledge and explanation about brainstem death. Franz *et al.* (1997) and DeJong *et al.* (1998) found that an understanding of brainstem death often affected relatives ability to donate organs, found generally poor understanding of brainstem death among both donating and non-donating families; and most particularly among non-donors. These studies found that relatives do need *appropriate* explanations of how clinical tests confirm brainstem death, and they should be given the opportunity to refuse attending brainstem-death tests.

Costain-Schou and Hewison (1999) wrote of the theoretical commitment among clinicians to 'truth telling', but also the operational assumption that individuals don't want to hear or won't understand technical details of illness and treatment. They found that there was a need for more openness and better information about the shape and meaning of treatment plans. While professional care providers need to be aware of the diverse concerns among families and the need to individualize information to each family's needs I suggest that, in the broadest terms, information so delivered has the potential to engender in families a sense of confidence that helps to give them the ability to care, to remain in control, and to find mechanisms to cope with their circumstances.

The lack of knowledge about brainstem death does indicate a need for education of both health professionals and the public. It is assumed that it could also be an issue for families with brainstem-dead relatives whose ventilator support is terminated and who do not become organ donors. Being given a chance to understand the information about the circumstances and time of death may also be an important issue for all bereaved families.

Conflict and resolution in donation decisions

Acute crisis may often put the carer in the situation of having to make decisions on behalf of their loved one. Conflict continued for participants throughout the process of decision-making about donation, deciding if donation should take place, and which organs or tissues should be donated. Decision-making to reduce conflict in the context of organ donation fits the criteria of complex decision-making. Among other features, Orasanu and Connolly (1993) suggest that an important characteristic of a complex decision problem is the uncertainty experienced by those involved in the resolution. Relatives who were unsure of the wishes of the deceased (or even if they possessed explicit knowledge of their wishes) were faced with a number of concerns.

Conflicts and resolutions for relatives concerning donation were about fulfilling the pre-mortem wishes of their loved one and assumptions about contributing to their perceived posthumous suffering, concerns that were conceivably exacerbated by a poor understanding of brainstem death or affected by the notion of *harming the dead* (Callahan 1987). Callahan (1987) highlighted the sentiment that it is possible to feel sorry for the dead person because we *do* think of the dead, as they were ante-mortem. Therefore, it is possible to experience compassion for the dead and to feel genuine moral outrage at broken pre-mortem promises, which fail to respect the wishes of the dead.

Relatives expressed two main concerns about donation, which were the mutilation of the body, and the possible suffering the donor might sustain as a result of the operation:

> I didn't know that it was an actual operation or anything, I just had these horrible visions of you know, sort of, you know, like a piece of meat, you know, stuck, dash and get it out and done with . . . like I say my visions was messy and all slap-dash business.

It was very important to participants that retrieval was carried out with dignity, propriety, and with utmost care and gentleness. They found the knowledge that retrieval was carried out as a proper surgical procedure reassuring:

> They say they do it so neat, especially for babies and small children, you can't even see the stitches, they do it so neat and tidy, that was such a lot of reassurance . . . .

There was another type of suffering that participants worried about. They felt that the potential donor had already suffered so much, a horrible death and invasive medical procedures. Was it fair to subject them to further indignities by allowing their organs to be removed? They were concerned about the vulnerability of their loved one at retrieval.

Relatives had to depend on information given to them by medical and nursing staff. It is worth considering the pressure that may have been implicitly exerted on relatives, in terms of the type of information and its timeliness to fit in with the overall prevailing atmosphere within the ICU at the time. The atmosphere could have depended on the workload and the degree to which staff shared in the philosophy of providing care for patients who were not likely to recover. Lipshitz (1993) highlighted the importance imposed by environments in which decisions are made, both in terms of understanding the decision and the strategies followed, which are influenced by the perceptions of the decision-maker.

So how did relatives make their decisions? Batten and Prottas (1987), Franz *et al.* (1997) and DeJong *et al.* (1998) noted that families would donate before completely coming to terms with their relative's death or precise understanding of brainstem death. Batten and Prottas (1987) suggest that being willing to act on the intellectual knowledge of death without its emotional acceptance may be what makes donation possible at all. Indeed, as suggested by Burroughs *et al.* (1998) and Whittaker (1990), it would raise the question as to whether more relatives may have consented to organ retrieval than would do so were they not in a state of emotional distress.

Decisions about donation were mainly consensus family decisions. Four main resolutions helped participants in their deliberations. These were the knowledge of the donor's wishes, the attributes of the donor, a personal realization of death, and confirmation of brainstem death. Personal motivations, such as wanting the life of the donor to continue, also played a part in participants' willingness to facilitate donation.

Participants' personal values also affected their ability to facilitate donation. For instance, some families placed importance on the quality of life of the individual and had sympathy for the lifestyle of people on dialysis, or were motivated by their commitment to the advancement of scientific knowledge. Some relatives felt that donation offered them an alternative to consenting to shut the ventilator down. Relatives who were asked felt that they probably would not have thought of organ donation and were glad they were approached. They felt it would have been distressing not to be able to fulfil the pre-mortem wish of the donor.

Callahan (1987) points out that the express wishes of the dead generally merit respect in their own right. This may help to explain the gratitude that was felt by relatives who were asked about donation and were able to facilitate the wish of the donor; a finding supported by Pelletier (1993b). It was also shown by Tymstra *et al.* (1992), Pelletier (1993a) and Douglass and Daly (1995), that knowing that they had made a worthwhile contribution, comforted relatives. Therefore, because of the importance attached to the wishes of the dead, and the action that relatives are able to take on their behalf, it seems imperative that next-of-kin should be given the option to facilitate donation. Surveys suggest that families want to be asked about donation (Manninen and Evans 1985). While Finlay and Dallimore (1991), Pelletier (1993b) and Featherstone (1994), report the distress caused when families were denied this opportunity. Relatives felt that their loved one's organs had been wasted and that they were denied the opportunity to have some good come from their loss. Pelletier (1993b) showed that relatives requested that health professionals should identify their relative as an organ donor; broach the subject of organ donation with them; discuss which organs and tissues they could donate; and acknowledge their wishes to donate.

Little is known about the choice to donate organs and tissues in other areas of health care. A case in point is organ and tissue donation within palliative care settings. How often is choice and decision-making restricted by not offering the option of tissue or organ donation to patients, and relatives upon the patient's death? Spivey's (1998) study about organ and tissue donation in palliative care found that in response to her questionnaire to 55% ($n = 83$) of palliative care matrons in England, it was found that 40% of units felt organ and tissue donation was appropriate, 21% felt it was inappropriate, and 39% did not know or gave reasons for not participating. Of the 40% of units that felt donation was appropriate, only two units requested routinely. The rest of the units only participated when a patient or family made the first enquiry.

Importance is, therefore, attached to the propriety of organ retrieval. It needs to be stressed during interaction with relatives, as well as in public education programmes; as there was misunderstanding among relatives about the nature and outcome of the procedure, which often led to disturbing fantasies:

> I just kept thinking if they lifted up the blanket, what would they find.

A daughter-in-law speaking of her experience of seeing her father-in-law after retrieval.

An appreciation of the historical influences and cultural values attached to the treatment of the dead (Richardson 1989) needs to form part of the theoretical underpinning of health professionals' education about donotransplantation. Health care professionals also need to reflect on their own feelings about the culturally perceived, unpleasant aspects of donotransplantation, to be more effective in giving or facilitating care of donors and their significant others.

With regard to decision-making, little is known about the way in which decisions are reached within the family group, and the responsibility families feel when making decisions on behalf of a relative who is moribund or newly dead. What are the processes of negotiation? What constrains the supremacy of the sick individual's desires? How much is weighted on the pre-mortem wishes of the relative and the desire not to harm the dead, or contribute to their perceived posthumous suffering?

Conflict and resolution in saying goodbye

Acute illness crisis that ends in unexpected death robs carers of opportunities for anticipatory grief, and may lead to poor bereavement outcomes. A lack of time and preparation before the death of the loved one may create difficulties in carers' ability to relinquish sentience that is attached to the body. This can create problems for carers in accepting death and 'saying goodbye' to the loved one. Opportunities also arise that may lead to hasty, ill-construed decisions about 'saying goodbye' or making arrangements for post-mortem care and the disposal of the body (Bradbury 1999). Such decisions could have consequences that affect the way carers are able to manage their bereavement and indeed may have a continued effect on the rest of their lives.

An opportunity to say 'goodbye' and share in the final moments of a loved one's life, has been documented by several authors to be important to many, and deep resentment can be felt among families when it was perceived that such an opportunity had been denied (Seale and Kelly 1997). Therefore recognition and an awareness of dying become important. Yates and Stetz (1999) identified five major categories with regard to families' awareness and response to dying:

- ◆ 'being uncertain' is the context where the carer may experience an ambiguous and unpredictable illness trajectory;
- ◆ 'agonizing' is a category characterized by emotional conflict of losing a loved one, watching their deterioration, and making life and death decisions about the continuation or discontinuation of treatment;

these were managed by:

- ◆ 'hoping' or reframing their experiences to envisage a positive future;
- ◆ 'pretending' choosing not to act as though the relative is going to die; and
- ◆ 'preparing' where they acknowledge the possibility of death and make public and private preparations.

Recently, research interest has been gathering momentum to elicit what it is that health professionals use as criteria to diagnose impending death. With the importance invested in the families' concern to be present at the deathbed, this area of investigation is becoming increasingly important.

Once organ donation was agreed, there came a time when relatives had to 'say goodbye'. This created further conflict and difficulty for relatives, in equating death with the appearance of the relative when making the decision to leave them. In no case did hospitals offer relatives a full range of options of visiting the relative post-retrieval, such as back on the ward, which might have been appropriate for some. This did cause regrets among relatives as they felt viewing the newly dead would have been preferable than, sometimes, days later at a funeral home. Retrospectively, relatives wished that they had more guidance from the hospital about options and the possible effects of choosing how and when they said goodbye. When this advice was given relatives were very grateful. A young mother reports:

> She [nurse] said to me, she said, 'Do you want to hold him?' I said, 'Oh, I don't know.' She said, 'Many people that don't hold their babies regret it later on . . . . Why don't you hold him?' I said, 'Oh, I don't know,' and she reassured me that you know, it was the best thing to do. So I did and I can't thank her enough, I am so glad that I held him for that last time, held him twice actually, in that same night, and I am so glad that I did, I think she is right, I would have regretted it not holding him for that last time . . . . I felt so chuffed, I felt so proud, my baby . . . .

Post-retrieval visiting with the body was shown to be important to some relatives as a means of helping them accept the death. As reported by the father who witnessed the brainstem-death test of his son:

> Father: The following day we went to the Chapel of Rest, we went in saw A there, there we saw . . .

> Mother: And there we saw a body freezing cold.

> Father: We saw death itself, which was a contrast, it was a stark contrast to what I had seen in the brainstem-test situation, that A hadn't looked cold and pallid and dead, he looked very much alive, but I had seen that he wasn't, but it underlined to me what the machine had, what the machine was actually doing for him, that the O_2 going in that made him look alive.

Seeing the body in its socially accepted form of deadness as a help to participants agrees with Worden's (1991) notions of the therapeutic value of deadness. However, this was a regrettable experience for other participants who felt unsupported and without adequate choices to say goodbye.

I suggest that it would be helpful for relatives to have the support of a nurse with them during this experience (preferably one they knew), from the unit where the donor received care. It would give the nurse a chance to view the body first and make sure it was in an acceptable condition to be visited. For instance, if eyes had been removed, that the face looks as natural as possible, this being important to relatives:

> Even though his corneas had been removed his eyes were carefully, his lids were carefully closed up and tiny stitches within the eyelashes which were hardly visible unless you really peered at them, and apart from that there were no other signs that anything [had been] removed.

Nurses could tell the relatives what to expect in terms of the setting in the Chapel of Rest, and what the donor might look like. Coupe (1991) stated that relatives said they were not given enough advice about how the body would look (particularly, with major organ donors, who will be very pale, due to the exsanguination of virtually their entire blood volume). Such interaction could also be helpful to nurses, as they would then be able to complete the cycle of nursing care, shown to be desirable for job satisfaction (Borozny 1990; Watson 1991).

Cultural expectations did have an impact on the aesthetic presentation of the dead body (Bradbury 1999; Verble and Worth 2000), which could be assumed to be particularly important, as the donors were relatively young. Participants had mixed feelings about the presentation of their relative after death. In some instances, they were satisfied by the way head injuries had been aesthetically presented:

> They done a marvellous job with the make-up at the undertakers, he just looked as if he was sleeping.

Others were very disappointed. A father said:

> The undertaker didn't even do him very well for us, that was another thing that really upset me, we went to see him, and to see him, he was all white wasn't he, his head, he was like Frankenstein wasn't he? I thought they would have covered up the wound so we wouldn't have seen it . . . . But it was strange to look at him and I kept thinking to myself, well you're not all there, there are parts missing . . . . Now, I think the worst bit was, that's the bit I remember most, is the, these clamps [in the head], I can still see them.

Overall, it appears that undertakers could consult more with families about their expectations: how they had last seen their relative (i.e. with or without head bandages); and what would be socially acceptable to them. It is especially important with donor families, as many donors have sustained head injuries, or operations, or their features have been damaged due to injury, or the effects of hospitalization. Health care professionals have a unique contribution to make in avoiding further damage to the features, by using their skills while caring for the patient; carrying out corneal recovery; and giving information to undertakers about anticipated problems in the presentation of the body.

'What do I do now?'

When leaving the hospital, some participants clearly felt abandoned, which is supported by Johnson (1992) and Finlay and Dallimore (1991). It was a confusing time leaving hospital and trying to come to terms with their changed situation. Participants often felt, 'A door had closed behind us'. They had very little support from the hospital with regard to their bereavement or transplant services to do with the donation. A wife told me:

> MS: When you left the hospital on the afternoon of the [date], do you remember if the hospital gave you any advice about grief or gave you any addresses of people that you might contact if you needed help or anything like that at all?
>
> Wife: They didn't give me anything.
>
> MS: Nothing at all?
>
> Wife: No, they just said, 'Cheerio, thank you very much for all you have done,' and away we went. That was it. They just said, 'Cheerio'.

A mother also explains the needs of her family at this time (Sque and Payne 1996, p.1366):

> We came away from that hospital with no support, nothing, just a plastic bag with his belongings in, nowhere where you could get in touch with anyone if you needed any counselling . . . . It's like you just walk away, empty you know . . . . If only they could find a nicer way of doing it, rather than just writing out a death certificate and sending you away with a plastic bag.

As much as participants in this study feeling lost and bewildered left an Intensive Care Unit, after a short relationship with staff had asked, 'What do I do now?'. An understanding is needed of the impact for families severing protracted relationships with health care professionals after a period of chronic illness or palliative care involvement.

Conflicts and resolution in the bereavement process

Conflicts continued for participants throughout their bereavement process. These conflicts concerned the incompatible notions of the continuance of the life of the donor with the reality of their death. Participants also wished their relative's contribution to be recognized, valued, and not forgotten. They clearly required continuing information and follow-up about the recipients that confirmed the achievement of the donor, such as the difference that the organ had made to the quality of their lives. Resolutions to these grief-conflicts were provided when information was available to participants about the outcome and continued contribution of the donation. Even if transplants failed, participants tended to feel that at least help had been offered. Could it be that information about recipients provided donor families with a sense of reassurance, which comforted them in the knowledge that somehow their loved one's organs had found a safe home again and there was now an integrated human wholeness that made the mutilation worthwhile?

One of most important things about donation and bereavement was that donation did not appear to affect the nature of grief but it changed the emphasis of death to focus on the donor's achievement, which demonstrated that kindness and caring continued. A father describes his feelings following his son's donation (Sque and Payne 1996, p.1366):

> It's not a reward that you get, it's something that happens as a result of a loved one wishing to give their organs to somebody else. They give their organs to somebody else so that they can have the gift of life and what they give to us is almost not an easy road in grief but a different road through grief, a less harsh road, and a less final death, because it is a death filled with different emotions, it's filled with the joy of knowing good has come out of his death, as opposed to us having to know that, just, ah, nothing has come out of his death, only pain and sorrow and sadness and also knowing that it is not only the recipient that receives, its their family, their friends . . . . It is a tremendous thing, it ripples out to hundreds of people . . . . Almost unending the relief and saving of pain that just giving something that is not needed can produce.

A lack of skilled bereavement support and pertinent information appeared to compound participants' distress. At the time of the interview, none of the participants regretted their donation decisions. It was important that participants felt they had made a contribution, through the right decision.

Contemporary bereavement theories may provide a way of interpreting loss but none of them account for the difficult choices that were made about shaping the course of that loss, and its outcomes, which were part of participants' organ donation experience. Stage theories of bereavement conflict with, and fail to embody, the notion of continuance (as part of the donor lives on), as bereavement is viewed as a process of recovery and resolution (Kubler-Ross 1969; Parkes 1972; Bowlby 1980; Worden 1991). Nor does the idea of a continuance after death abide comfortably with our culturally assumptive world of deadness. Problems also arise in trying to interpret the post-donation experience using Walter's (1996) theory for survivors to form a durable biography of the dead person, when part of them is perceived to continue living. Boss (1991) suggested (within the constraints of *boundary ambiguity*) such a lingering; unfinished bereavement can be extremely difficult for relatives.

Furthermore, the normal boundaries between the acceptance of loss, and attachment to the deceased individual and their body, may be complicated by the knowledge that part of the deceased lives on, or that their donation has been life-preserving, or life-enhancing for another. How does this fit with the development of Walter's (1996) and others durable biography of the dead and the role of the organ recipient? Clearly we are dealing with an irreconcilable tension. For these families the recipient has become part of the donor's biography, 'living on'. This may help to explain donor families continuing interest in recipients' welfare, as well providing support for the bonds that were felt to exist between them, and the sentience attached to the organ.

Klass *et al.* (1996) have suggested that what bereavement researchers have observed are people altering and continuing their relationship with the dead person. They propose that it is normative for mourners to maintain a presence and connection with the deceased and that this presence is not static. Remaining connected seems to facilitate an individual's ability to cope with the loss and accompanying changes in their lives. These connections provide solace, comfort, and support, and ease the transition from past to future. Survivors construct a sense of the deceased and develop inner representations of them. People are changed by the experience of bereavement, they do not get over it. Part of that change is transformed by continuing a relationship with the deceased. The talk of biography (Walter 1996) may also help the restructuring of the donor's life in the process of adaptation and change in the post-death relationship of new connections. Therefore information about recipients needs to be viewed as contributing to the increased capacity for the bereaved to resolve grief conflict by playing some part in helping to complete the biography of the decedent (Walter 1996). Within the constraints of confidentiality, the continued benefits and value of the transplant, over time, could be communicated to relatives.

What about the experience of bereavement in other contexts of chronic illness? Following an exhaustive review of the literature I was forced to draw the conclusion that after having made the commitment to support families in their bereavement the research was at least ambiguous, whether palliative care provided any protective effect for families or impinged upon their bereavement. This raises issues about the efficacy of palliative care intervention. Seale (1989) suggested that such outcomes need to consider the adoption of palliative care principles in hospitals and the possible use by hospice staff of more traditional systems of care. There needs to be more research to refine and improve the quality and credibility of palliative care in this regard.

Conclusion

This chapter has described a study that suggested that relatives' experience of organ donation could be explained by a theory of 'dissonant loss'. During the donation process conflict existed for relatives in two particular forms. On the one hand, conflict existed as a series of events over which they had no control, such as the ambiguity of brainstem death. Other conflicts emerged through decisions that needed to be made about donation. These decisions tended to take place in a highly charged emotional environment. The theory suggests areas where help may be focused and may usefully be applied to other situations of loss that involve conflicts and complex decision-making, such as in mutilating elective surgery, termination of treatment, or discontinuing life-support.

Concern is often expressed about the best way to support family members in these situations but the best way to do this is not always clear because of the dynamic nature of the terminal illness trajectory, and the caring and changing roles of the people caught within it. Understanding family experience in our plural society needs much hard work as factors such as race, ethnic identity, gender, kinship relationships all play a part in how individuals understand, interpret, and fulfil their roles during the terminal trajectory. Further development needs an appreciation of the complexity of human need and intra-family relationships.

References

Batten, H. L. and Prottas, J. M. (1987). Kind strangers: the families of organ donors. *Health Affairs*, 6, 35–47.

Borozny, M. (1988). Brain death and the critical care nurse. *The Canadian Nurse*, 84, (1), 24–27.

Borozny, M. (1990). Codman award paper—the experience of intensive care unit nurses providing care to the brain dead patient. *AXON*, 12, (1), 18–22.

Boss, P. (1991). Ambiguous loss. In *Living beyond loss: death in the family* (ed. F. Walsh and M. Goldrick), pp. 165–175. W.W. Norton & Company, New York.

Bowlby, J. (1980). *Attachment and loss 3: loss sadness and depression*. The Hogarth Press, London.

Bradbury, M. (1999). *Representations of death: a social psychological perspective*. Routledge, London.

Burnhill, R. (1999). A study of anticipatory grief in an Italian population: 'A journey of hope.' MSc thesis. University of Surrey.

Burroughs, T. E., Hong, B. A., Kappel, D. F., and Freedman, B. K. (1998). The stability of family decisions to consent or refuse organ donation: would you do it again? *Psychosomatic Medicine*, 60, 156–162.

Callahan, J. C. (1987). Harming the dead. *Ethics*, 97, 341–352 .

Costain-Schou, K. and Hewison, J. (1999). *Experiencing cancer: quality of life in treatment*. Open University Press, Buckingham.

Coupe, D. (1991). A study of relatives' nurses' and doctors' attitudes of the support and information given to the families of potential organ donors. MPhil thesis. University of Wales.

DeJong, W., Franz, H. G., Wolfe, S. M., Nathan, H., Payne, D., Reitsma, W. *et al.*(1998). Requesting organ donation: an interview study of donor and nondonor families. *American Journal of Critical Care*, 7, (1), 13–23.

Douglass, G. E. and Daly, M. (1995). Donor families' experience of organ donation. *Anaesthesia and Intensive Care*, 23, (1), 96–98.

Featherstone, K. (1994). Nurses' knowledge and attitudes toward organ and tissue donation in a community hospital. *Journal of Trauma Nursing*, 1, (2), 57–63.

Field, D. (1993). Care for relatives of brain stem dead patients going for organ donation. *Care of the Critically Ill*, 9, (2), 72–74.

Finlay, I. and Dallimore, D. (1991). Your child is dead. *British Medical Journal*, 302, 1524–1525.

Franz, H. G., Dejong, W., Wolfe, S. M., Payne, D., Reitsma, W., and Beasley, C. (1997). Explaining brain death: a critical feature of the donation process. *Journal of Transplant Coordination*, 7, (1), 14–21.

Fulton, J., Fulton, R., and Simmons, R.G. (1987). The cadaver donor and the gift of life. In *Gift of life: the effect of organ transplantation on individual, family, and societal dynamics* (ed. R. G. Simmons, S. K. Marine, and R. L. Simmons), pp. 338–376. Transaction Books, New Brunswick.

Glaser, B. and Strauss, A. (1967). *Discovery of grounded theory*. Aldine, Chicago.

Jasper, J. D., Harris, R. J., Lee, B. C., and Miller, K. E. (1991). Organ donation terminology: are we communicating life or death? *Health Psychology*, 10, (1), 34–41.

Johnson, C. (1992). The nurses' role in organ donation from a brainstem dead patient: management of the family. *Intensive and Critical Care Nursing*, 8, 140–148.

Klass, D., Silverman, P. R., and Nickman, S.L. (1996). *Continuing bonds: new understandings of grief*. Taylor & Francis, Washington.

Kubler-Ross, E. (1969). *On death and dying*. Macmillan, New York.

Lawton, J. (2000). *The dying process: patients' experiences of palliative care*. Routledge, London.

Lipshitz, R. (1993). Converging themes in the study of decision making in realistic settings. In *Decision making in action: models and methods* (ed. G. A. Klein, J. Orasanu, R. Calderwood, and C. E. Zsambok), pp. 103–137. Ablex Publishing Corporation, Norwood, New Jersey.

Manninen, D. L. and Evans, R. W. (1985). Public attitudes and behaviour regarding organ donation. *Journal of the American Medical Association*, 253, (21), 3111–3115.

Molter, N. C. (1979). Needs of relatives of critically ill patients: a descriptive study. *Heart & Lung*, 8, (2), 332–339.

Orasanu, J. and Connolly, T. (1993). The reinvention of decision making. In *Decision making in action: models and methods* (ed. G. A. Klein, J. Orasanu, R. Calderwood, and C. E. Zsambok), pp. 3–20. Ablex Publishing Corporation, Norwood, New Jersey.

Parkes, C. M. (1971). Psycho-social transition: a field for study. *Social Science & Medicine*, 5, 101–115.

Parkes, C. M. (1972) Bereavement: studies of greif in adult life. International University Press, New York.

Parkes, C. M. and Brown, R. (1972). Health after bereavement: a controlled study of young Boston widows and widowers. *Psychosomatic Medicine*, 34, 449–461.

Parkes, C. M. (1993).Bereavement as a psychosocial transition: processes of adaptation to change. In *Handbook of bereavement: theory, research and intervention* (ED. M. Stroebe, W. Stroebe, and R. O. Hansson) pp. 91–101. Cambridge University Press, Cambridge.

Pelletier, M. (1993a). Emotions experienced and coping strategies used by family members of organ donors. *Canadian Journal of Nursing Research*, 25, (2), 63–73.

Pelletier, M. (1993b). The needs of family members of organ and tissue donors. *Heart & Lung*, 22, (2), 151–157.

Richardson, R. (1989). *Death, dissection and the destitute*. Penguin Books, London.

Savaria, D. T., Rovelli, M. A., and Schweizer, R. T. (1990). Donor family surveys provide useful information for organ procurement. *Transplantation Proceedings*, 22, (2), 316–317.

Seale, C. (1989). What happens in hospices: a review of research evidence. *Social Science & Medicine*, 28, (6), 551–559.

Seale, C. and Kelly, M. (1997). A comparison of hospice and hospital care for people who die: views of surviving spouses. *Palliative Medicine*, 11, 101–106.

Shanteau, J. and Linin, K. A. (1990). Subjective meaning of terms used in organ donation: analysis of word associations. In *Organ donation and transplantation psychological and behavioural factors* (ed. J. Shanteau and R. J. Harris), pp. 37–49. Washington, American Psychological Association.

Spivey, M. (1998). *Organ/tissue donation within palliative care settings*. BA dissertation. University of Luton.

Soukup, M. (1991). Organ donation from the family of a totally brain-dead donor: professional responsiveness. *Critical Care Nursing*, 13, (4), 8–18.

Sque, M. (1996). The experiences of donor relatives, and nurses' attitudes, knowledge and behaviour regarding cadaveric donotransplantation. Ph.D. thesis. University of Southampton.

Sque, M. (2000). Researching the bereaved: An investigator's experience. *Nursing Ethics*, 7, (1), 23–34.

Sque, M. and Payne, S. (1996). Dissonant loss: the experiences of donor relatives. *Social Science & Medicine*, 43, (9), 1359–1370.

Sykes, N. P., Pearson, S. E., and Chell, S. (1992). Quality of care of the terminally ill: the carer's perspective. *Palliative Medicine*, 6, 227–236.

Tymstra, Tj., Heyink, J. W., Pruim, J., and Slooff, M. J. H. (1992). Experience of bereaved relatives who granted or refused permission for organ donation. *Family Practice*, 9, (2), 141–144.

Verble, M. and Worth, J. (2000). Fears and concerns expressed by families in the donation discussion. *Progress in Transplantation*, 10, 48–55.

Walters, A. J. (1995). A hermeneutic study of the experiences of relatives of critically ill patients. *Journal of Advanced Nursing*, 22, 998–1005.

Walter, T. (1996). A new model of grief. *Mortality*, 1, (1), 7–25.

Watson, K. (1991). Developing positive attitudes to procurement surgery. *ACORN Journal*, 4, (6), 31–36.

Whittaker, M. (1990). Bequeath or burn? *Nursing Times*, 86, (40), 34–37.

Worden, W. (1991). *Grief counselling and grief therapy: a handbook for the mental health practitioner*. Routledge, London.

Wright, B. (1996). *Sudden death: a research base for practice* (2nd edn). Churchill Livingstone, New York.

Yates, D. W., Ellison, G., and McGuiness, S. (1990). Care of the suddenly bereaved. *British Medical Journal*, 301, 29–31.

Yates, P. and Stetz, K. M. (1999). Families' awareness of the response to dying. *Oncology Nursing Forum*, 26, (1), 113–120.

Chapter 7

Family caregiving: a gender-based analysis of women's experiences

Christina Lee

Family caregiving, the home-based care of ill or disabled family members, is a responsibility that falls disproportionately on women (Hooyman and Gonyea 1995; Schofield *et al.* 1997). Surveys from Australia (Schofield *et al.* 1997), the USA (Miller *et al.* 1991), and the UK (Wenger 1994) suggest that around 75% of caregivers are women, while the gender bias is even greater in Japan (Tokyo Metropolitan Government 1995). In the current economic and political climate, public support for the disabled and frail is inadequate (Hooyman and Gonyea 1995), and the responsibility for this burden falls increasingly to the family. This arrangement may appear less costly than the provision of adequate social services, but only because the costs to the caregivers are not considered (Finch and Groves 1983; Osterbusch *et al.* 1987).

Research on the impact of caregiving focuses on 'caregiver burden', demonstrating that caregiving has significant negative impacts on emotional health (e.g. McNaughton *et al.* 1995), physical health (e.g. Schulz *et al.* 1990), and quality of life (e.g. Schofield *et al.* 1997). Caregiving also restricts the caregiver's capacity to participate in other social roles; reductions in leisure time (e.g. Miller and Montgomery 1990) and employment opportunities (e.g. Abel 1991; Wagner and Neal 1994; Schofield *et al.* 1997;) affects economic status, as well as opportunities for personal development and social interaction (Abel 1991; Hooyman and Gonyea 1995). An Australian survey of caregivers (Schofield *et al.* 1997) found that 27% of respondents were spending over 100 h weekly in caregiving and a further 15%, between 31 and 100 h.

The majority of research on family caregiving focuses on the individual experiences of family caregivers and fails to take broader social factors into account. Lee (1999) has argued that this individual focus has obscured the social and cultural forces underlying the fact that the majority of family caregivers are women, and thus has allowed researchers and policy makers to ignore the gender inequities which are perpetuated by an assumption that family caregiving is naturally the work of women. The burden of caregiving is not insignificant, and there is a need for analyses and interventions that address issues of public policy rather than the individual woman and her personal ability to cope.

Hooyman and Gonyea (1995) have argued that family caregiving provides an illustration of the way in which arduous and socially necessary work is absorbed by women and then rendered invisible through invocation of women's 'natural' ethic of care. This chapter uses quantitative and qualitative analyses of the impact of family caregiving in the lives of Australian women to demonstrate the burden of family caregiving and to illustrate the gender-based assumptions that maintain the inequitable distribution of this important but under-recognized work.

The Women's Health Australia project

Women's Health Australia is a longitudinal survey of the health of Australian women, funded by the Australian Commonwealth Department of Health (Brown *et al.* 1996). Three cohorts of Australian women, in three age groups (18–23, 45–50, and 70–75), were recruited in 1996 through the records of the Health Insurance Commission, which holds data on Australia's universal health care system, provided to all citizens and permanent residents. Selection was on a stratified random basis, on place of residence (urban/rural/remote), with deliberate over-sampling from rural and remote areas, where women were selected in twice the proportions of the Australian population living in these areas. Approximately 42 000 women have responded to the survey, which is projected to continue for 20 years, to provide a longitudinal perspective of influences on the health of Australian women. The survey, which will be repeated on a 3-yearly cycle, includes over 250 closed-response questions, including measures of quality of life, health care usage, satisfaction with health care services, health-related behaviours, and demographics. This paper discusses responses to both closed- and open-ended questions dealing with family caregiving, using the data provided in 1996 by women in the 45–50 (middle-aged) and 70–75 (older) groups. Rather than comparing women with men, the aim of the project is to understand the factors that influence the health and well-being of women from their own perspective; thus, this chapter focuses exclusively on women's experiences.

Participants

A total of 13 888 women in the 45–50 age group responded to the 1996 survey, a response rate of 56% to an unsolicited mail survey. Their mean age was 47.8 years, with 82.6% married or in stable relationships. Fifty per cent had completed 10 years of education, 37% had completed 12 years of education or had a trade certificate or diploma, and 12.5% had a university degree. In the 70–75 age group, 11 939 women responded, a response rate of 40%. Their mean age was 72.6 years, with 57.1% married and 34.4% widowed. Thirty-eight per cent had completed 10 years of education, and 27.5% had 12 years or more. Comparisons with census data indicate that these samples are demographically representative of the Australian population of women in this age group (Brown *et al.* 1998).

Family caregivers: quantitative aspects

A total of 1775 middle-aged respondents (7%) and 1235 older respondents (10%) answered two questions about family caregiving ('Do you regularly provide care or assistance, e.g. personal care, transport, to any other person because of their long-term illness, disability or frailty?' and 'Are you happy with your share of the following tasks and activities: caring for another adult who is elderly, disabled or sick?') consistently to indicate that they were caregivers.

Data from this sub-group of women were compared with the remainder of the sample in order to address the following questions:

- description—who they are;
- who they care for;
- the effects of caregiving on employment, finances, physical and emotional well-being, coping, and leisure, and social activities.

Socio-demographic variables included marital status, education, employment status, place of residence (urban, rural or remote), living arrangements, and a subjective rating of ability to manage on her income. Physical health was rated through a single global item, as well as by ratings of experience of a range of common symptoms such as backache and difficulty sleeping. Respondents also reported whether they had been hospitalized in the previous year, and how often they had visited a general practitioner, medical specialist, or other health professional for their own health in the previous year. Health behaviour was assessed through self-reports of smoking, alcohol use, and participation in mammography and cervical screening.

Well-being was assessed with the physical and mental summary scales of the SF-36 (Ware and Sherbourne 1992). In addition, respondents were asked how often they felt rushed or pressured, how often they had spare time on their hands, and how stressed they felt. Other variables that were not measured quantitatively emerged from qualitative analysis.

Family caregivers: qualitative aspects

The final page of the 1996 survey was headed with the request, 'Have we missed anything? If you have anything else you would like to tell us, please write on the lines below', and the remainder of the page was left blank for comments. After transcription and preliminary coding of all responses, 185 middle-aged women and 168 older women were identified as having mentioned caregiving for family members (comments on caring for one's own children or grandchildren were not included in this analysis, unless the child was described as experiencing a physical or emotional problem).

A series of questions was derived from a review of the empirical literature on family caregiving (Lee 1999), leading to a focus on specific issues. We wanted to know who the respondents cared for and what they did for those people, in order to gain an overall picture of their objective situations. We also wanted to know the effect of caregiving on employment and finances; physical and emotional well-being; coping strategies; and leisure and social activities.

Data analysis

Statistical comparisons were carried out between caregivers and others on responses to closed questions, and transcribed comments were subject to content analysis.

Following this analysis, comments that were not readily encompassed by the themes identified by the existing empirical literature, were examined and a third set of questions, based on emerging themes, was identified.

Findings

Who cares?

The quantitative analyses indicated few demographic differences between caregivers and others. Among the middle-aged, caregivers did not differ from non-caregivers in age, marital status or education, but were significantly less likely to live in remote areas (4.4% vs 7.1%, d.f. = 2, χ^2 = 17.86, $P < 0.001$) and more likely to share a house with their parents (14.3% vs 2.4%, d.f. = 1, χ^2 = 512.0, $P < 0.0001$), adult relatives (4.6% vs 1.9%, d.f. = 1, χ^2 = 43.35, $P < 0.0001$), or another person's children (5.5% vs 3.7%, d.f. = 1, χ^2 = 11.00, $P < 0.001$). Older caregivers did not differ from non-caregivers in age, area of residence or education, but were significantly more likely to be currently married (71% vs 56%, d.f. = 2, χ^2 = 112.4, $P < .001$).

Who do they care for?

Open-ended descriptions indicated that caregiving could be highly complex, with 50 middle-aged women (27%) and 15 older women (9%) caring for two or more different people, often in different locations.

Middle-aged women were most likely to care for their own disabled children (44%), parents and parents-in-law (41%), or husbands (18%). Older women were most likely to care for their husbands (69%), with 15% caring for adult children and 8% caring for their mothers, all of whom were well into their 90s. Other women cared for aunts and uncles, siblings, disabled grandchildren, and close friends.

The women described a wide range of disabilities and illnesses experienced by their family members; their children frequently experienced physical or intellectual disabilities, emotional and psychiatric problems, and chronic physical diseases such as cerebral palsy or epilepsy. Parents of the middle-aged women, and husbands and mothers of the older women, were described by many respondents simply as frail or in need of care, but they also reported a range of severe medical conditions, the most common being stroke, Alzheimer's disease, cancer, and Parkinson's disease. Many of these older family members had multiple problems. The husband of one older woman, for example, suffered from prostate cancer, emphysema, and Alzheimer's disease; another had cancer, a stroke, and Parkinson's disease.

While the rhetoric of family- or community-based care tends to be based on the assumption that a co-operative family group will share the care of a single member in need, the evidence (e.g. Max *et al.* 1995) suggests that most caregiving is carried out by a single family member. Further, several respondents to this survey described complex situations in which a single caregiver was trying desperately to support several generations of her family without any assistance. One middle-aged woman wrote:

> Have husband with major heart-lung problems . . . 23 year old son with Cystic Fibrosis . . . 19 year old son with acute brain injury (due to MVA [motor vehicle accident]) . . .

mother-in-law 90 yrs who needs to be taken to doctors . . . . Coped until I had MVA 4 years ago and then our life has just seemed to have a major collapse. Have had to put farm on market due to illness of family.

What does caregiving involve?

The middle-aged women generally described their caregiving in vague terms, if at all (e.g. 'care and help'). Typical descriptions came from a woman who provided 'support with transport to specialists, etc., household maintenance, and general care' for her ageing parents, and another who wrote, 'My time is spent caring for a child with Cystic Fibrosis—home, physio, medication, hospital visits—in- and out-patient, help with education access, etc.'.

Some older women described nursing duties such as: 'give daily injections . . .'; '. . . I help to change his stoma every 4 days . . .'; 'rubbing liniment on his aches and pains'. Some mentioned housework (e.g. 'Most days I cook lunch for a friend of mine who has cancer but still lives in his own home') or financial activities (e.g. 'my husband is in care due to Alzheimer's disease so I have to pay the bills and I also see him nearly every day'). One woman whose husband's 'mental condition has deteriorated' commented positively on the change in her role: 'I now do things that I didn't think I could do in my younger years—the finance, driving and managing, in our case the farm'.

Caregiving for institutionalized family members

The caregiving literature tends to assume that the decision to move a dependent relative into professional care, while it may be a difficult one, will mean an end to caregiving and to the stresses associated with it (e.g. Gold *et al.* 1995). This, however, was not the case for many of the older women, several of whom wrote about their continued sense of responsibility for husbands or mothers in care. Some certainly did see institutionalization as a relief from burden. For example:

I cared for [husband with stroke] for 9 years at home until 10th August 1995, when he went into a nursing home because I could not care for him at home any longer owing to his immobility. Caring for him over such a long period had a very wearing effect on me physically and my concentration, etc. were affected. I am now getting back to my normal self and feeling much better.

Others, however, seemed to have internalized the ethic of care to the extent that they felt guilty or distressed that they were no longer able to provide home-based care. For example:

I think that the stress and trauma resulting from the sale of our home, the subsequent relocation to a unit and the grieving which has taken place since my husband's admittance to the nursing home, have exacerbated my health problems.

I have my mother 95 in a Nursing Home which I find hard to cope with because there is so little I can do.

Alzheimer's disease has far reaching effect on carer! [husband] is now in care—The feeling of stress exists still (or is it guilt).

Yet others found that their family member adjusted poorly to institutionalization and made them feel guilty. As one elderly woman wrote:

> My husband is in Nursing Home since December 28 last year and he is not adjusting and is always complaining about it and can't understand why he can't be at home or just visit. It's impossible to make him understand it's not my fault because he is a big man and can't walk—needs two to three men to lift him and this house has steps and I am not well enough to look after him 48 hours a day. Can't get him to the toilet or bathroom in and out of car. He can't even stand up and is getting worse. He gets very cross with me and upsets me as I can't think how I can help him to be more content, and I have been told not to visit him every day and spare myself all of the stress he gives me. But I feel bad if I don't go to see him as no one else will visit him because of his manner. Crying and upsetting them.

The extent to which women internalize their caregiver role is demonstrated by the fact that many continued to play a major role in their institutionalized family member's lives, visiting regularly:

> My husband is a permanent resident at local nursing home suffering from advanced Alzheimer's disease and Parkinson's disease. I visit him every second or third day.

> . . . I am able to see him [husband] every day and can take him out in a wheelchair.

or bringing their family member home for frequent visits:

> My husband . . . is currently in a nursing home but I bring him home at least five days a week for between 2–6 hours. Other days I visit him in the home. I do this because he is confined in the dementia ward with 20 other patients, none of whom are able to speak. My husband is still able to converse and although he doesn't read very much he is still interested in the outside world.

In many cases, they continued to carry a significant burden of practical care:

> I have my husband who is terminally ill with brain tumour in Nursing home and find it hard to come to terms with, having to visit each day to feed him, etc.

> I am stressed at this time as my husband is in hospital with Parkinson's Disease and is in poor health. I will most days, do his washing and feed him if needed, so I don't have a lot of time to relax and do things I'd like to. I miss him and spend a lot of the day with him.

Employment and finances

Questions about employment were analysed for the middle-aged group only, as very few of the older women had paid employment. The quantitative data showed that fewer of the middle-aged carers were employed on a full-time basis (26.6% vs 36.1%; $\chi^2 =$ 95.89, d.f. = 2, $P < 0.001$) than the comparison group. Nevertheless, 19.2% of carers (compared to 22.4% of non-carers) worked more than 40 h per week in addition to their caring responsibilities. Middle-aged carers were significantly more likely to report finding it either 'impossible' or 'difficult' to manage financially (48.6% vs 43.1%, d.f. = 1, $\chi^2 = 18.27$, $P < 0.0001$), but there was no difference among the older group.

The qualitative data from the middle-aged women supported these findings. The assumptions that middle-aged women do not need or want employment, and that their financial needs are provided for by husbands, were not supported by these respondents. Careers, employment, and finances were strained and in many instances respondents were unable to seek paid employment or were forced to leave satisfying careers. For example:

> I had to leave school at a young age due to my mother's poor health .... I would still love to learn a lot more but due to my both parents' ill health my time is very limited between visits to my parents, which is every other day.

> I have not been able to work because of [multiply handicapped adult child], as there is not any child care centres to have children of special needs in the school holidays once they are past school age.

Combining work and caregiving was an option for some women, though this appeared difficult to manage, and several respondents described a sense that their caregiving role interfered with their ability to perform well at work. For example:

> I often find the stress/lack of sleep affects my diabetes and this in turn occasionally affects the level of my work as an RN and I feel that I am not functioning to my full capacity, and could maybe at some time lose my job. It is not mistakes in my work just the fact that I am working much slower than others at times and I lose confidence in myself.

Some of those who were unable to work in paid employment reported that finances were strained by the reduced income and by increased family expenses associated with caregiving. The following quotes illustrate the range of financial pressures that arose:

> We are both on Invalid Pension (me wife's) and I receive a domiciliary nursing care benefit. But this still doesn't cover our needs. One, we are paying off a mortgage; there goes most of one pension pay. Our expenses are more than a normal pensioner without disabilities, wheelchair, shoe repairs and medication, therapy aids demand a part of our finances, plus normal home and car insurance/maintenance etc. We can't afford home care.

> ... the housing told me bluntly to use our money first, which is $25,000 but won't last for ever, out of our pension we pay $420 per fortnight for rent, the shopping, electricity, phone, MBF [health insurance] so every month we have to go to the bank, this gets me down, looking after my husband day and night and money worries. Always paid our tax never been in debt, never ask for anything till now, but nobody listens but when the money is gone so will we because living on a pension is the last straw. I have seen what it does to people.

> ... If the village increases the monthly levy again, I will have to give up the car.

Physical health and psychological well-being

The quantitative data indicated that middle-aged carers had poorer health than their counterparts, while this was not so for the older group. Middle-aged carers were significantly more likely to report their overall health as being 'fair' or 'poor' than non-carers (14.4% vs 11.1%, d.f. = 1, χ^2 = 16.63, $P < 0.001$), and more likely to report back aches, joint problems, chest pain, breathing difficulties, indigestion and constant tiredness.

Among the middle-aged women, there was no difference in the number of visits to either a general practitioner, medical specialist, or other health practitioner over the course of a year. The older carers reported fewer visits to general practitioners (22%

had attended fewer than three times in the previous year, and 25% more than seven times, compared with 19% and 31% of the non-carers, d.f. = 3, χ^2 = 18.35, $P < 0.001$) and fewer visits to specialists (81% had attended fewer than three times, compared with 76% of non-carers, χ^2 = 16.60, $P < 0.001$), but did not differ from non-carers on visits to other health professionals. The middle-aged carers were significantly more likely than others to have been admitted to hospital within the 12 months prior to the survey (18.6% vs 16.2%, d.f. = 1, χ^2 = 6.70, $P < 0.01$), while the older caregivers were less likely (20.6% vs. 23.3%, d.f. = 1, χ^2 = 4.64, $P = 0.03$). These data suggest that the middle-aged women were experiencing negative physical effects from caregiving, but that, if anything, the older caregivers were perhaps in slightly better health than those who did not provide care. This may be because older women in poor health may be relieved of caregiving through the institutionalization of their family members, while those who continue in good health are expected to continue to provide care.

Middle-aged caregivers scored significantly lower than non-caregivers on the physical component of the SF-36 (means 48.6 and 49.7; $F = 21.48$, d.f. = 1, 13 886, $P < 0.001$), but there was no difference for the older women (means 50.2 and 50.0). On the mental component of the SF-36, carers scored lower than non-caregivers in both age groups (middle: means 45.6 and 47.3, $F = 30.43$, d.f. = 1, 13 886, $P < 0.001$; old: means 49.0 and 50.7, $F = 30.7$, d.f. = 1, 10 387, $P < 0.001$). Carers experienced significantly greater stress than non-carers in both age groups (middle: means 8.01 and 6.52, $F = 118.9$, d.f. = 1, 13 766, $P < 0.001$; old: means 4.00 and 2.67, $F = 200.0$, d.f. = 110 356, $P < 0.001$). Both middle-aged and older carers were significantly more likely to report feeling busy, rushed or pressured (middle: 64.5% vs 60.6%, d.f. = 1, χ^2 = 9.68, $P < 0.005$; old: 40.3% vs 20.6%, d.f. =1, χ^2 = 247.4, $P < 0.001$), and less likely to report having time on their hands (middle: 9.5% vs 12.3%, d.f. = 1, χ^2 = 11.45, $P < 0.001$; old: 8.5% vs 14.0%, d.f. = 1, χ^2 = 28.3, $P < 0.001$). Thus, there was consistent evidence that both middle-aged and older caregivers experienced poor emotional health and high levels of stress.

Examination of the qualitative data suggested that the caregivers generally saw their physical and psychological health as irretrievably intertwined, and assumed that the emotional stress of caregiving would lead inevitably to physical illness. Typical quotes from middle-aged women were:

> . . . disability . . . in the family . . . affects everyone. It's exhausting which must in turn affect one's health.

> . . . at present I attribute my eating problems, overweight, chronic depression, sleeping problems and fatigue, to problems associated with my son's disability.

> . . . [caring for ex-husband] resulting in myself recognising being in depression and seeking help. I am currently on antidepressant medication and am at present reducing the dose with a view to ceasing in time. Taking control of own health! Last week I had a cholecystectomy. I feel was a physical manifestation of the stress levels I experienced . . . .

The older women were more likely to describe themselves as being in 'reasonable physical health for my age', but suffering physically and emotionally. They interpreted symptoms such as tiredness and aches and pains as inevitable aspects of ageing, but also felt that these symptoms increased the difficulty of caregiving and caused increases in stress and depression. One woman, whose husband was institutionalized, epitomized this perspective:

> The days I bring him home I find very stressful as he is very demanding. At 75 years of age with osteoarthritis of the spine I find pushing my husband around in the wheelchair and often showering and dressing him very tiring.

Other elderly women reported developing physical problems as a result of caregiving. For example:

> . . . for 12 months I was helping my friend 80 years old to shower and dress her (she had broken her elbow and shoulder bone). I pulled a muscle in my neck since then have been to physio, X-rays, specialist. They say it is arthritis and strained neck.

Other older women commented that they were too old to provide the care that was expected of them, but did not seem to expect that anybody else would take the responsibility in their place:

> I don't wish to complain but at 70 years the going is hard at times.

> I am almost 73 years of age and past being a carer.

Health behaviours and preventive health activities

Middle-aged carers were significantly more likely to report being current smokers (20.9% vs 18.1%, d.f. $= 1, \chi^2 = 8.05, P < 0.005$), but less likely to drink alcohol more than once a week (35.2% vs 40.2%, d.f. $= 1, \chi^2 = 15.73, P < 0.001$) than non-carers. Older carers and non-carers did not differ in smoking status (5.9% and 5.7%) or drinking more than once a week (28.0% and 29.5%). Among the middle-aged women, there was no difference in the proportion having mammograms within the past two years (53.1% vs 52.6%). Carers were, however, significantly less likely to have had a Pap smear within the last 2 years (67.5% vs 71.5%, d.f. $= 1, \chi^2 = 11.36, P < 0.001$).

While none of the middle-aged women mentioned preventive health behaviours in the open-ended section, several of the older women mentioned the impact that caregiving had on their ability to maintain their own health. Several mentioned that they were unable to be as physically active as they would like:

> I am a great walker and up to two years ago I had no trouble walking to the city and back. As I now look after my 98 year old mother I do not have the time.

> I am fortunate to have very good health but now, being virtually house bound and social life almost non-existent, I feel that my health will surely deteriorate.

Others commented on reduced or disrupted sleep:

> My husband has Parkinson's Syndrome in the early stages. He is 80 years old . . . . He is very restless at night so neither of us get proper sleep.

> . . . my sleep is so interrupted most nights that I feel tired next day.

Thus, while there is no evidence to suggest that the older caregivers are more likely to suffer from major illness, they certainly are stressed and tired, and concerned that the burden of care will affect their own health. At the same time, however, they seem to accept this as an inevitable consequence of their roles as wives and daughters.

It is worth emphasizing that, of course, men also take on the role of caregivers and, when they do, generally have similar experiences to those of women (e.g. Kaye and Applegate 1990). However, over 70% of caregivers in Australia and the UK are women (e.g. Wenger 1994; Schofield *et al.* 1997), with even greater gender disparity in other countries (e.g. Tokyo Metropolitan Government 1995). However, neither men themselves nor representatives of health care services seem to assume that it is 'naturally' men's role to care, with even men who are engaged long-term in the care of family members believing that women are somehow more appropriate to the task (Kaye and Applegate 1990).

Coping strategies

The focus on the individual, which is apparent in research on caregiver burden, is also apparent in interventions that aim to relieve this stress. Much of this work focuses on improving the coping strategies of individual women in order to reduce health care costs (e.g. Gallagher-Thompson and DeVries 1994; Peak *et al.* 1995). Interventions do not generally attempt to challenge the broader social structure that places intolerable demands on a powerless, frequently elderly, and overwhelmingly female section of the community. It has been argued (e.g. Abel 1987) that such a perspective on the problem, which aims to help unpaid family carers to accept and adjust to a role in which they have no personal freedom and no opportunity for change, is in fact teaching them to connive in their own exploitation.

Some respondents did discuss their own personal coping resources, frequently expressing pride that they had coped with situations that they found extremely difficult. Middle-aged women wrote:

> I found there was very little assistance readily available to assist in coping and that I had to find huge resources of time, energy, and emotional strength within myself.

> I can now feel proud I was strong enough to cope apparently in one piece.

Older women expressed similar sentiments:

> I have found a strength that I didn't know I had.

> I've survived—I'm fantastic.

> Have bandages in bathroom, kitchen, and car shed—never a dull moment. Coping with both I usually just take the line of least resistance and light another cigarette. I don't think I really know the meaning of stress. Some people who talk about stress is just an ordinary day to me.

More commonly, though, the middle-aged respondents in particular described a combination of personal, family, social, financial, and religious sources, which helped them cope, as illustrated by the following quotes:

> Fortunately my health is good. I have a supportive spouse and children and we are very fortunate that we can cope [financially] in spite of the fact that my income has been diminished . . . .

Luckily our family unit is very strong—and we have all helped our son through a very difficult time.

. . . all the hard work was a success and [daughter with leukaemia] is now 21 and happily married. The thing I'm trying to say though is you can have the best medical help available but without the love and support from a loving family and friends you will not survive.

Social groups and hobbies helped some respondents to cope, for example:

I have a love of craft and belong to a Patchwork Group. The support and help this group has given me has been invaluable. Sharing a common interest with other women in a great stress reliever.

My part-time job and weekly art class help my emotional and mental health enormously. I also try to retain a good sense of humour in situations and this attitude tends to relieve stress.

Spiritual or religious beliefs were mentioned as a source of strength by three women:

We are a Christian family and try to build our lifestyle on Christian principles and seek God's guidance in our daily lives. When we consider others more, 'self' falls into a better perspective and I am amazed at how God really does provide!—even to our adopted children!

The older women, like the middle-aged women, identified a range of strategies and supports that helped them to cope. Family and friends were important sources of support, but for these older women it seemed more likely that family members were too busy to help. Thus, while some considered themselves to be well supported, others saw themselves as having to cope without family support:

I care for invalid husband, I have daughter living with me who is very helpful.

My family are very supportive but work keeps them busy.

The other four of my children all live and work in Sydney, Melbourne and Perth and all have families of their own so unable to help me very much But generally I cope fairly well and can't really complain. Just at times I feel a little lonely but busy myself and garden, etc. Soon feel better.

Time out

The literature identifies leisure activities and time out as important in helping caregivers to cope, and in support of this perspective one elderly woman wrote:

3 years ago my husband was knocked down by a car . . . a change of life style has been necessary to cope with things such as his short term memory loss, circumscribed social life, lack of concentration, physical dependence, etc. Last month when he has at last been able to be left relatively on his own (with help from family and friends) I have had a month's holiday backpacking in ancient sites in Turkey. This time completely away has given a great rejuvenation to my health, both mental and physical.

However, many older women were unable to take even short breaks from caregiving. A common theme was a sense of regret that caregiving meant they had no time for themselves and no opportunities for relaxation or enjoyment. Again, however, women seemed to accept that this was an inevitable result of their personal circumstances, not the result of social policy. Many mentioned restrictions on social activity (e.g. 'At present caring for husband with terminal illness therefore unable to take part in social activity'; 'Our social activities have changed greatly because of my husband's health and I care for him which is a 24 hour commitment'). Others regretted having little time for hobbies, interests, and charity work: 'I have given up all voluntary work'.

Several older women expressed a wish to take time off or spend more time on themselves but appeared to accept that this was entirely impossible:

> My husband is very demanding and I would love to have a holiday away from him for just a couple of weeks, but placing him into somebody else's care is virtually impossible.

> I am reasonably fit but am unable to pursue outside interests due to my husband needing constant attention. He has a degenerative disease. Also he is unwilling to have respite care, and that makes it very difficult for me to have any outside interests. I used to do marching also voluntary work at hospice.

For some women, restriction on discretionary time had been a major and life-long challenge. As one elderly mother of two disabled sons wrote:

> Support services in the community were practically non-existent, so the bulk of my life or most of my energy has gone into coping with them. One did not ever walk and lived until he was almost 22 and the younger one is still alive—but did not walk until he was nearly nine years. My life has depended on my fitting enough interesting activities around these problems.

Exploitation and the ethic of care

Awareness of the 'ethic of care' was expressed in two complementary ways by these respondents. While some women, particularly in the older age group, appeared to have internalized this ethic, others perceived it as imposed against their will by broader social systems, which were hostile to their personal needs, and expressed a sense of betrayal or exploitation.

The older women seemed most likely to have internalized a sense that it was their natural role in life to take on the care of the disabled. Many wrote positively about their relationships with disabled spouses and described themselves as grateful to be able to support their husbands. For example:

> The two of us have been looking after each other with our nervous breakdowns and have come through OK. He looked after me all those 30 years especially those first few years when I was so bad he was so attentive. He still is to this day. It's been my turn to look after him now. He has just had 3 operations in 4 months and could have a stroke anytime so we make the most of each day and look after each other.

> I am 74 years of age. My husband is 91. He suffers from acute angina and needs care but can care for himself such as dressing bathing, helping a little, such as wiping up, setting table. My eldest son shall be 56 in August. He is confined to a wheelchair. He has never walked. He is a person with cerebral palsy. The only thing he can do for himself is feed himself. I care for him at home, and happy to do it. I have a good family. I believe in taking each day as it comes, and I thank God he has given me good health to be able to care for John and Jim.

In 1990 my husband had major surgery for bowel cancer . . . attended the cancer clinic for 5 years. During all this I was able to look after him and help him with everything. He also has trouble with his legs and has ulcers on his legs and I've been able to dress these and see to them also. Two years ago I had major surgery for Diverticulitis which complicated with other problems, collapsed lung, etc. and my husband looked after me for over 18 months until I was well again. I'm explaining this to you to let you know how myself 74 years old and my husband 79 years old, and married 57 years now and still able to look after each other and thoroughly enjoy doing it. Thank you.

Not all the descriptions of contented mutual caregiving in old age were completely consistent with the rosy Darby and Joan image that some women seemed to want to project. For example:

My husband has required Nursing Home care for the last 12 months. He has Dementia due to strokes. I visit him at least 4 to 5 times a week and when weather is suitable, take him out for walks. He seems to enjoy the outing, but not always does he know me. These are very special times for us, as we have had a very special 51 years of marriage. I do his laundry, I feel one of the remaining things I can do for him. His sickness has been evident for 14 years. I was sad when last year I was beginning to 'crack' from the strain of the demands of such an illness.

By contrast, middle-aged women were more likely to express openly the sense that family caregivers were making a valuable but unappreciated contribution to the country's health care system:

I do the work of an occupational and physiotherapist, nurse, housewife, psychologist, chief cook and bottle-wash, gardener and finance manager and for that I receive $57 a fortnight, $28 a week. It's cruel that 'carers' have so little value in the Government's eyes. My job as carer is 24 hours a day every day with no respite, no holidays and yet I'm saving the Government thousands of dollars as are many other carers because we do CARE. We've been in situations where there's not been enough money to buy food and we've had to live on what meager items were in cupboard.

The sense that responsibility fell inequitably on female family members was addressed directly by some respondents. For example:

I find a lot of my stress is due to my parents . . . . My parents seem to think that I should be there for them always. They make you feel guilty. I have 3 brothers—but everything is left up to me.

Caring for a child like [intellectually disabled son] places enormous stress on a woman— In my case it probably was in part responsible for marriage breakdown and I've found that you really become the sole parent of a child like this. Since separation my ex-husband has not had anything to do with the disabled child.

Conversely, the carer ethic for some women was strong enough that they felt they had no choice but to continue to support their husbands, no matter what the circumstances. For example:

. . . my husband told he had a terminal illness. I found that hard to cope with. But 2 years ago, my daughter Suzie, told me my husband had sexually abused her as a child. Major to cope with. There was a lot of help for her but not much for me or my husband. I felt I couldn't leave because of his illnesses and two other children to care for. My physical and mental health were very low. Our marriage was very unsteady.

An older woman felt obliged to provide care even though she felt ill suited to the task:

. . . at the moment have a lot of responsibilities as my husband is wheelchair bound and I am his carer. I don't feel it is the right job for me as I get impatient with him and feel guilty as it is not his fault he is the way he is . . . . I feel stressed and tired a lot because I feel very responsible for my husband's well being and safety.

Several older women, without explicitly blaming a social system that pressures older women into caregiving, described deep distress over the turns that their lives had taken For example:

At times I feel very drained and trapped in a situation over which I have no control. I want to be as supportive as I can and I think my own health is suffering as a consequence.

I do not feel stressed, although sometimes I feel bad-tempered at the way life has turned out for me at a time when I could have looked forward to a comfortable retirement.

One middle-aged woman summarized the consequences of the 'ethic of care' for women as follows:

After spending more than three quarters of your life raising kids—looking after a husband—friends—relatives—other people's kids—full time care of your elderly mother—divorcing—selling—moving house—building—kids leaving home—sudden death of your parents and mother—who you've looked after full time for years—bad relationships—when the partner can't stand you speaking to your kids, etc. One morning you wake up completely exhausted—Everything's gone. And you wonder—'Who the hell are you?' and where am I supposed to go from here? And why do women—mostly—give so much time of themselves doing for others—and never taking some time out for themselves—or even given some thought to—one day it might all disappear—everyone else gets on with their lives and you're left wonder[ing] where to start again—or if you've even got or care to have the strength to do so.

Discussion

The quantitative and qualitative data presented here illustrate the need for a gender-based analysis of family caregiving. The difficulty and complexity of many caregivers' situations demonstrates that family caregiving is not always the only imposition on an otherwise tranquil life. Women are more likely than men to experience ill health and psychological distress (Lee 1998), more likely to cope with multiple and conflicting roles (Christensen *et al.* 1998; Doress-Worters 1994), and less likely to be well off in terms of finances, education, and career (e.g. Australian Bureau of Statistics 1997). Caregiving responsibilities must be seen in the context of contemporary women's lives, and sexist assumptions about women's natural place in the family need to be avoided in seeking solutions to this growing social problem. In particular, the assumption that all women are naturally suited to caregiving and will always be able to find the personal and financial resources to cope with the needs of a family member must be questioned by the evidence presented here.

The quantitative data show that caregivers experience poor mental health, are limited financially and in employment opportunities, and feel stressed and overworked. Interestingly, the middle-aged caregivers seem to be in poor physical health while the older women are in relatively good health. This may result from older women in poor health being more able to access professional health care for their family members.

The qualitative data present a picture of women coping with difficult situations with little practical support. The middle-aged women describe restrictions on employment opportunities, concerns about their own physical health, and a sense of abandonment and exploitation by the health and social security systems. The older women, reflecting the more traditional gender-role attitudes of women in their age group, appear more likely to have internalized the ethic of care, to the extent that a large number see no alternative to full-time caregiving, even when they recognize their own needs for rest or time out; and many continue to care for family members even after they have been institutionalized. Others interpret difficult personal circumstances as simply what should be expected at their age, or describe their arduous lives in positive terms as an opportunity to demonstrate their lifelong devotion to family members.

The findings of this study, although cross-sectional, provide further evidence of the dilemma being faced by women who take on a caregiving role in a society that provides no acknowledgement and very little support for this significant family role. Family caregiving has clear economic benefits to the wider community. When older people live with their adult children, their use of formal services is reduced (Choi 1994) and this reduces expenditure at a public level. The fact that this is at the expense of those families, and particularly of the women in those families, is often ignored.

Government agencies and employers alike continue to see caregiving and its conflicts as primarily a private issue and a 'women's problem', which is not relevant to employment conditions or the provision of health and welfare services (Gonyea and Googins 1992). However, health agencies need to recognize the burden of caregiving and provide carers with adequate practical and financial support. The existence of genuine choices through adequate provision of full- or part-time nursing care, either in institutions or through home-based systems, would undoubtedly be a considerable financial expense at a public level, but would provide the frail and disabled, and those people who currently care for them, with genuine choices and remove the inequitable burden that currently falls on a predominantly elderly and female group (Hooyman and Gonyea 1995). Current policies, which are based on a consideration of direct public expenditure to the exclusion of all other factors, such as the appropriateness of the care to the individual, serve to maintain social and gender inequity (Sommers and Shields 1987).

Provision of public services should be combined with adequate financial support for family caregivers, including acknowledgement and support of the travel needs of frail people and their caregivers who live in isolated areas. Such a change to public policy might increase the extent to which caregiving became a genuine choice, and might serve to change the perceived balance between the burdens and satisfactions of caregiving.

Qualitative research is useful in providing a richness of detail that is often lacking from quantitative evidence. These women's stories, overall, provide an impression of a group of women leading lives of quiet desperation, with a sense of having been abandoned by the society to which they provide a valuable service. They illustrate the importance of this growing health and social problem, and the need to seek solutions that go beyond individuals and beyond the assumption that women are always, naturally, available to care for family members without payment or assistance.

References

Abel, E. K. (1987). *Love is not enough: family care for the frail elderly.* American Public Health Association, Washington.

Abel, E. K. (1991). *Who cares for the elderly? Public policy and the experiences of adult daughters.* Temple University Press, Philadelphia.

Australian Bureau of Statistics. (1997). *Australian women's yearbook 1997.* Australian Government Publishing Office, Canberra.

Brown, W. J., Bryson, L., Byles, J., Dobson, A. J., Manderson, L., Schofield, M. *et al.* (1996). Women's Health Australia: Establishment of the Australian longitudinal study of women's health. *Journal of Women's Health,* 5, 467–472.

Brown, W. J., Bryson, L., Byles, J., Dobson, A. J., Lee, C., Mishra, G. *et al.* (1998). Women's Health Australia: Recruitment for a national longitudinal cohort study. *Women and Health,* 28, 23–40.

Choi, N. G. (1994). Patterns and determinants of social service utilization: comparison of the childless elderly and elderly parents living with or apart from their children. *Gerontologist,* 34, 353–362.

Christensen, K. A., Stephens, M. A. P., and Townsend, A. L. (1998). Mastery in women's multiple roles and well-being: Adult daughters providing care to impaired parents. *Health Psychology,* 17, 163–171.

Doress-Worters, P. B. (1994). Adding elder care to women's multiple roles: a critical review of the caregiver stress and multiple roles literatures. *Sex Roles,* 31, 597–616.

Finch, J. and Groves, D. (ed.). (1983). *A labour of love: women, work and caring.* Routledge and Kegan Paul, London.

Gallagher-Thompson, D. and DeVries, H.M. (1994). 'Coping with frustration' classes: development and preliminary outcomes with women who care for relatives with dementia. *Gerontologist,* 34, 548–552.

Gold, D. P., Reis, M. F., Markiewicz, D., and Andres, D. (1995). When home caregiving ends: a longitudinal study of outcomes for caregivers of relatives with dementia. *Journal of the American Geriatrics Society,* 43, 10–16.

Gonyea, J. G. and Googins, B. K. (1992). Linking the worlds of work and family: Beyond the productivity trap. *Human Resource Management,* 31, 209–226.

Hooyman, N. R. and Gonyea, J. (1995). *Feminist perspectives on family care: policies for gender justice.* Sage Publishers, Thousand Oaks, CA.

Kaye, L. W. and Applegate, J. S. (1990). *Men as caregivers to the elderly: understanding and aiding unrecognised family support.* Lexington, MA: Lexington Books.

Lee, C. (1998). *Women's health: psychological and social perspectives.* Sage Publishers, London.

Lee, C. (1999). Health, stress and coping among women caregivers: a review. *Journal of Health Psychology,* **4**, 27–40.

Max, W., Webber, P., and Fox, P. (1995). Alzheimer's disease: The unpaid burden of caring. *Journal of Aging and Health,* 7, 179–199.

McNaughton, M. E., Patterson, T. L., Smith, T. L., and Grant, I. (1995). The relationship among stress, depression, locus of control, irrational beliefs, social support, and health in Alzheimer's disease caregivers. *Journal of Nervous and Mental Disease,* 183, 78–85.

Miller, B. and Montgomery, A. (1990). Family caregivers and limitations in social activities. *Research on Aging,* 12, 72–93.

Miller, B., McFall, S., and Montgomery, A. (1991). The impact of elder health, caregiver involvement, and global stress on two dimensions of caregiver burden. *Journal of Gerontology,* 46, S9-S19.

Osterbusch, S., Keigher, S., Miller, B., and Linsk, N. (1987). Community care policies and gender justice. *International Journal of Health Services,* 17, 217–232.

Peak, T., Toseland, R. W., and Banks, S. M. (1995). The impact of a spouse-caregiver support group on care recipient health care costs. *Journal of Aging and Health,* 7, 427–449.

Schofield, H. L., Herrman, H. E., Bloch, S., Howe, A., and Singh, B. (1997). A profile of Australian family caregivers: Diversity of roles and circumstances. *Australian and New Zealand Journal of Public Health,* 21, 59–66.

Schulz, R., Visintainer, P., and Williamson, G. M. (1990). Psychiatric and physical morbidity effects of caregiving. *Journals of Gerontology,* 45, P181-P191.

Sommers, T. and Shields, L. (1987). *Women take care: The consequences of caregiving in today's society.* Triad Publishers, Gainesville, FL.

Tokyo Metropolitan Government. (1995). *Living conditions of the elderly.* Tokyo Metropolitan Government, Tokyo.

Wagner, D. L., and Neal, M. B. (1994). Caregiving and work: consequences, correlates, and workplace responses. *Educational Gerontology,* 20, 645–663.

Ware, J. E., and Sherbourne, C. D. (1992). The MOS 36-Item Short-Form Health Survey (SF-36): I. Conceptual framework and item selection. *Medical Care,* 30, 473–483.

Wenger, G. C. (1994). Dementia sufferers living at home. *International Journal of Geriatric Psychiatry,* 9, 721–733.

Chapter 8

The contribution of carers to professional education

Frances Sheldon, Pauline Turner, and Bee Wee

Introduction

Earlier chapters have shown that carers have many needs, which go unrecognized by professionals in health and social care. This highlights the importance of giving professionals a broader education to support them in their attempts to deliver the best care and support to someone who is seriously ill. The perspectives of carers have been a focus throughout this book, and are now being incorporated into new approaches to qualifying and postqualifying professional education. In this chapter, we examine what carers may bring to the education of professionals, reviewing research and practice in this area, and describe a five-year education project. We argue that there is considerable potential for developing carers' contributions. We suggest guidelines for good practice that will enable the full value to be gained from what they can offer.

Why invite carers to contribute to professional education?

The weight placed on the carers' contribution to both care and education may depend on the underpinning philosophy of that particular field of health and social care. Patients have always been involved in the area of professional education. However they have traditionally played a relatively passive role in acting as the teaching 'material' or focus for learning. There is now an increasing trend towards recognizing the patient as an active resource and participant in education (Hendry *et al.* 1999; Stacey and Spencer 1999). Hajioff and Birchall (1999) suggest that it is helpful to view the patient as both 'consumer' and 'subject', in their paper advocating the use of outpatient clinics as a learning setting. Wykurz (1999), in his commentary on patients in medical education, suggests the notion of 'citizenship' in exploring the potential contribution patients can make in medical education.

Whether in a passive or active role, patients have always received far more focus from students in the health care professions than their carers have. These students will always have encountered carers in clinical settings, but have not necessarily been enabled to recognize their contribution as part of the educational process. An emphasis on the bio-medical approach and on the disease, with the patient as the focus of attention in much health professional education, is a key influence here, though this is changing. Paediatrics, for example, is an area where carers, usually parents in this case, are recognized as having an equal role alongside professionals, and where there are a number of initiatives involving carers in contribution to professional education. Blasco *et al.* (1999) describe their Parent-as-Teachers programme, where paediatric residents in Minnesota learn through home- and community-site visits about the importance of developing partnerships with parents and service providers in order to give better care to children with chronic conditions. This programme is in fact very similar to the Family Study programme at Southampton University, in which second-year medical students visit families with a newborn baby on several occasions to learn about child development and the impact of a new baby on the family. Social work education, embedded in the social sciences and humanistic counselling, underpinned by a commitment to equal opportunities, has always given the family and society more emphasis. For a social worker in a health care setting the client may frequently be the carer rather than the patient.

There are also the issues highlighted by Twigg and Atkin (1994) in their conceptualization of the range of ways that service agencies, and professionals working in them, respond to carers. If carers are valued largely in relation to what they can offer the patient, as 'resources' or 'co-workers', then professionals will only have a narrow focus on them in their caring role. Twigg and Atkin suggest that a stance from professionals, which supersedes or transcends the caring relationship and recognizes carer and cared-for as separate human beings with possible conflicts of interests, will produce a valued outcome that promotes independence for both parties and may support carers in aspects of their lives apart from the caring role. Meeting carers in person, hearing them tell their stories, is likely to have more force in promoting such a stance than simply reading case studies. We would argue that carers have an equal right to be considered 'citizens' alongside patients, and our own experiences show that carers can contribute significantly and helpfully to both the content and process of learning. In palliative care, our own area of practice, one of the key principles is that the person who is dying, and those who care about them, are the unit of care for professionals (National Council for Hospice and Specialist Palliative Care Services 1995).

In the UK, government policy now demonstrates a commitment to valuing carers' contributions in all areas of health and social care. This is evident from the passing of the *Carers (Recognition and Services) Act* in 1995, providing an entitlement to assessment of their ability to care for those giving 'regular and substantial care' and making it a duty for local authorities to take into account the carers' ability to care when looking at the support needed, and from the publication of *Caring for Carers*, the Government's national strategy for carers (Department of Health 1999). So far that trend has been felt most in the service sector but there is now the beginning of a recognition that professional education must follow suit if professionals are to be properly prepared to understand and value carers. The publication of the English National Board's document *Learning from Each Other* (ENB 1996) is an example. A recent edition of the CAIPE Bulletin (Vanclay 1996) describes some UK initiatives, mainly involving patients or clients rather than carers, though in a more recent edition a researcher can still lament that it is 'comparatively unusual for patients or non-professional carers to participate in interprofessional education' (Tope 1998, p.11).

Another factor encouraging carer contribution to education may be the recognition of the considerable reliance on carers in chronic illness. Family caregivers who are members of the Council of Relatives to Assist in the Care of Dementia (CRAC) have been providing sessions for students on a variety of courses training doctors, nurses, and psychologists in London since 1988 (Soliman and Butterworth 1998).In practice too, in palliative care patients become frail towards the end of their illness, clinical change occurs rapidly, and efforts to fulfil some patients' wishes by maintaining them at home as much as possible mean that it is not easy to arrange regular workshops with patient involvement. This was one of the pragmatic reasons for seeking carer's contributions to the undergraduate inter-professional workshops described below.

Different knowledges

Schön (1987) has described the complex and challenging world of professional prac-tice where 'messy, confusing problems defy technical solution'. In professional educa-tion, whether at qualifying or postqualifying level, students learn ways of dealing with this world, and both the process and content of the education may contribute to this. In any educative experience the teacher, the student, members of the student's group, the person needing a service, and their carer, may all contribute different facets of knowledge and experience to understanding and working with individual and unique situations, which also have something in common with other situations in the same field of care. In professional education, the teacher commonly has had practice experience at some stage to inform their now more theoretical and research-based emphasis. Students bring a variety of life experience, which even for younger students now encompasses the world of work and for health and social care students that work is often as an untrained care assistant. Models of learning that treat students as passive recipients of information, without recognizing that what they bring informs their learning, have no place in contemporary professional education (Coles 1996).

Carers have areas of knowledge, both about the person they are caring for and about their own caring activities and needs. Harvath and colleagues, from a study of the care of frail older people, have characterized the different types of knowledge that profes-sionals and carers bring to a situation as *cosmopolitan* and *local knowledge* (Harvath et al. 1994). *Cosmopolitan* or professional knowledge is based on a general understand-ing about a condition or situation derived from principles, theories, and skills learnt in training and developed through practice. The *local* knowledge they define as (Harvath et al. 1994, p.30):

> ... the skills and understanding that the family brings to the caregiving situation . . . . derived from experience in managing the older person's chronic illness and is embedded in the context of the family culture and relationships.

They argue that it is only by drawing on both types of knowledge that satisfactory care is likely to be provided. There is a parallel here in Barry and Henderson's study of terminally ill cancer patients in an oncology unit and decision-making (Barry and

Henderson 1996). They identified different ways of knowing of patient and doctor in relation to the disease. The doctor's way of knowing is grounded in scientific and factual data, whereas the patient's emerges from the lived experience of the disease—the local knowledge. As their disease progressed, patients built up their local knowledge and desired to be more, rather than less, active in decision-making than when admitted for the first time. In fact they perceived themselves to be less consulted. Barry and Henderson comment that the potential gap between actual and preferred decision-making widens because each party fails to communicate their expertise to each other.

Nolan *et al.* (1996) similarly endorse a view that carers are experts in their own situations with their knowledge of both the present position and of what has gone before. Of course the person who needs a service brings their own perspective, and it is well-established that their carer is not always a satisfactory proxy for informing professionals about their needs (Higginson *et al.* 1990). Perhaps Field and colleagues supply the solution here with their recognition that both carer and the person needing the service have legitimate but different viewpoints, which inform their accounts (Field *et al.* 1995).

However it is often professional knowledge that is privileged over local knowledge when decisions are taken about care. For example, a daughter caring for her mother was offered respite care at her local hospice. She told the admitting nurse about her mother's preference for sleeping with her pillows in a particular way to help her breathe more easily and to sleep better. When she visited her mother next day she found her mother looking very uncomfortable and complaining that she had been unable to sleep that night. Her daughter's local knowledge had been ignored. Why do professionals find it so hard to incorporate the carer's perspective? For some, doing so may be too challenging to their confidence in what they bring to the situation; for others there may be real or perceived conflicts between the carer's view and the view of the person needing the service. A nurse tutor working with CRAC commented on the fact that her interaction with a carer as a practitioner on the wards had a different focus from when carers came to teach on her course (Soliman and Butterworth 1998, p.27):

> When I was a ward sister I heard what carers had to say . . . . Why is it so different when they come to the ENB N11 Carers' Day? Because the power is different. As a ward sister I was assessing . . . starting to work out what sort of things I was going to provide because that is my role.

In other words, there might be a different value attributed to the knowledge that a carer brings into an institutional setting compared with when the carer is invited to contribute because of their local knowledge—a tendency to see carer's knowledge only as a contribution to the professional assessment and not in its own right, to regard them as a 'resource' in Twigg and Atkin's terms (Twigg and Atkin 1994) or a problem. In the example above, in the teaching situation, power was more equal and this enabled the ward sister to hear the carer's story in a different way and develop an emotional resonance with the carer present in person, which could not be gained from a text book.

Schultz *et al.* (1993) has suggested that a cognitive shift is needed to recognize the existence and value of different types of knowledge. There is clearly a challenge to professionals in first making that shift and then sustaining it while maintaining their professional contribution. We want to suggest that the one way to help this cognitive shift take place is to ensure that students on professional qualifying and postqualifying courses are assisted to value the contribution of carers. Here we draw on Eraut (1994) who proposes that professional knowledge is built up from many individual experiences both in formal learning and practice situations, and that as the student brings knowledge into a situation, that knowledge is developed and changed by working with it in the situation. We want to describe some work that supported students in such a process.

Case study: involving carers in undergraduate inter-professional training

We are drawing on our experience of witnessing first hand the contribution of carers to education from the interaction that takes place between them and undergraduate students. It is based on five years experience of running, each academic year, nine inter-professional workshops in palliative care at monthly intervals at Countess Mountbatten House, a specialist palliative care unit. These involve students from nursing, medicine, social work, physiotherapy, and occupational therapy from Southampton University. The workshops are facilitated by a consultant in palliative medicine, a lecturer in palliative nursing, and a social work lecturer in psychosocial palliative care, who are all members of the Education Team at Countess Mountbatten House with previous experience of collaborating in delivering clinical care.

A unique feature of these workshops is that family carers who are either recently bereaved or who are caring for someone with a terminal illness are interviewed by students. They are usually a partner but sometimes a parent, sibling, or offspring. They are not selected on any basis other than that they are willing to participate, nor are they trained. They are recruited by the clinical staff involved with the care of the person the carer is looking after. A member of the education team then telephones to explain the purpose of the session and what their contribution might be. Some carers contribute on more than one occasion and when this is so they often relate different aspects of the care received. However we aim to limit the number of separate occasions that a carer participates to a maximum of four. This is to maintain the sense of freshness for them and to avoid possible over-commitment through a sense of gratitude for the service they have received from the palliative care unit. Overall, it is impressive how many are not only willing to come and share their experiences but eager to 'give something back' so that students can benefit from them.

They tell powerful and personal stories, both good and bad, about the care that they, and the patient, experienced. The authenticity that these carers bring, and the experience of hearing about care from those who are at the receiving end, could not be communicated by the facilitators alone.

The format of the workshops has been carefully developed. During the first half, students work on specific tasks in small inter-professional groups in order to understand each other's training and to get to know each other. This enables students to begin to establish a sense of working together, which is essential preparation for the more risky task of interviewing the carer later in the morning. The students then meet the carer in the same small groups and work on another set of explicit tasks (Box 8.1) to help them understand the carer's experience. After the carer leaves, students feed-back their observations to the whole group. During this time there is opportunity to reflect on, discuss and check back issues raised by the carer's story.

Box 8.1 Interviewing the carer (Group task)

- Interviewing the carer.
- Briefly hear the carer's story.
- What different professionals were involved?
- How was their input co-ordinated?
- Who was the 'key' person who made (or didn't make) it work?
- What would have made it go better (for the patient, the carer, the other professionals)?

The facilitators often highlight aspects of the carer's story to broaden the learning experience, otherwise students can become overwhelmed by the emotion of one carer's story and fail to pick up the real lessons that should be transferable. The facilitators have a part to play in supporting the students and carers through the learning process. They recognize that hearing the carer's story is very powerful and may raise personal issues for students. They also recognize that the carers may need support through the experience. As a result, they ensure that carers come together both before and after they meet the students so as to have an opportunity to talk over any concerns, ask questions and 'debrief'. Often within a group there is at least one carer who has already been to a workshop and who is able to respond to questions and concerns from the others who are attending. Following the interview, the carers have opportunity to say what the experience has been like for them and to continue talking about issues that have been raised. We have observed that this is often a time when the carers appear to gain mutual support from chatting to each other and recounting their experience of looking after a family member or coping with bereavement.

What do students learn from carers?

In the evaluations of every workshop during the last five years, students comment on the value of meeting a carer, referring to it in terms of the 'impact' that it has had on them. They feel privileged at hearing the carer's story and learn an enormous amount about the experience of care-giving. It is interesting that students say they have not had the opportunity to meet family carers before. They may meet family members on hospital wards but they do not have the insight or the encouragement, it seems, to rec-ognize that these may be important people to talk to. It is clear, then, that having an opportunity to do so is of tremendous value to the students and enables them to see care in all its different facets through the carers' eyes, and pinpoint new and signifi-cant insights into care provision and their own professional response.

One important realization that students make is that carers are knowledgeable in their own right. However, the *nature* of this knowledge is different from that which the students have and may occur at different levels. For example, one carer, whose husband had a rare cancer, had become more knowledgeable about that cancer than most health professionals. The students recognized that it was important that professionals did not become defensive in this type of situation. Another carer recounted how adept she had become at helping her husband, who had a brain tumour, to be as independent as possible in mobilizing, washing, and dressing. She was constantly irritated when agency nurses, who came to do a night shift at her house, 'took over' the care without bothering to learn from her expertise. Carers often become expert in this way about the practical aspects of caring and they are, of course, usually knowledgeable about the person being cared for in a way that no professional carer could be.

On the other hand, students are surprised at the carers' lack of knowledge in other areas. For example, they lack understanding about medical terminology and are often ignorant about disease and disease processes, treatment, side-effects, and issues around prognosis. Carers' stories include many instances where patient and family needs change rapidly but the services they receive are not always flexible enough to meet those needs. The stories demonstrate that there is often a lack of knowledge about systems of care; for example, carers usually do not understand the interface between social services and health, and are often unaware of the issues surrounding policy and funding. As facilitators who hear family carers' stories again and again, we have gained a lot of insight into difficulties that many carers have in accessing 'the system'. Some only manage to do so if they have 'inside information', in other words they have a friend or relative who works in health or social care; others only do so after they have struggled with difficulties for some time or have reached crisis point. The clear message is that the system, which provides health and social care, must become more 'user-friendly' and easier to access. This is an important message for students to learn during their training, and evidence from an in-depth evaluation over three months (Coles *et al.*, in preparation) suggests that students were keen to learn in what ways they could improve things so that carers would not be let down in future by professionals and systems that were intended to provide help but which often failed to do so.

One of the constantly recurring themes is to do with communication. The students discover how to listen attentively without needing to ask the 'routine medical and nursing questions'. They hear of the lasting effects of how information about diagnosis and prognosis was given and thus learn at first hand about good and bad techniques in breaking bad news. They also learn that a chance statement or action on the part of the professional might have a lasting impact, for good or ill, on patient and family. They also learn that the family carer, like the patient, needs time. It is striking how many carers say that they have never had focused time in which to talk about their own needs. These are often overshadowed by those of the ill person.

Students also see the importance of good communication between professional colleagues. A key focus for the workshops is about inter-professional working and one of the questions, which we encourage the students to find answers to, is: 'how well do the professionals work together in providing the care that the patient and family receives?'. Several issues of importance have emerged from the stories that family members tell us:

- The importance of a keyworker. This may be any member of the team who has built up a rapport with the patient and carers. This is often a co-ordinating role in which the keyworker involves other professionals as the need arises and maintains an overview of the patient and family's care.

- The importance of 'hearing' what the person is saying and not jumping to conclusions or making assumptions.

- The importance of continuing to visit, even when there seems very little in the way of treatment that can be given. Carers often say how helpful and supportive it is when the general practitioner continues to visit, even though he or she may have little to offer in the way of medical advice.

The students appear to learn from all the carers' experiences, however negative some of them may seem. For example, students often show strong identification with their profession-to-be by taking responsibility for the sometimes poor quality of professional care provided. They feel a need to apologize to the carers for their particular professions. They want to ask in what way they could improve things so that carers will not be let down in future by professionals and health care systems that are intended to provide help but which often fail to do so.

Students also learn how to work together. Carers speak of rapidly changing clinical situations. Their stories are often harrowing and intense. Students who are not used to dealing with such situations rely on each other's support in order to elicit the story and to support the carer during the story-telling. They adopt a team approach naturally—as if the intensity of the real-life experience makes them cling together. The experience of 'being thrown in the deep end', as one student put it, can have positive outcomes for them and carers. Although the experience may evoke an emotional response in either students or carers, this does not feel like a weakness but rather an appropriate response to a real event.

Although hard evidence is required to show that this type of exposure leads to improved care, it is probable that the experience of meeting the carer will remain with the students. Indeed some of their comments suggest that it will have a lasting impact on practice. As Gibbs (1992) observes, 'The motivational content is established by the emotional climate of the learning'. The idea of 'negotiating' for patients and carers and of listening to them emerged from a comment made by one of the students as follows:

> The impact of today has changed me so much. I'm determined to listen to patients. We tend at work to do this and that, and then this . . . we are so busy. I will not be so 'clinical' but I will find out their [the patient and carer's] needs and talk to them more.

What do carers get out of being involved?

We felt it was important to find out from carers how they felt about the experiences of contributing to the undergraduate inter-professional workshops. Consequently, we invited them to participate in a group discussion at the end of one academic year in which they were able to talk about meeting the students (Turner *et al.*, 2000). From their comments, and also our experience over the five years, we can make some observations about what carers gain from taking part.

First, it is clear that the carers enjoy the opportunity to contribute to professional education. They value the opportunity to present a real-life experience to the students. One carer said:

> They need to be given experience of human feelings. When you train you become a robot—they [health care staff] put you down this lane as if you do this, you do that, you do the other. You've got to do this by a certain date and they forget that you aren't just a number. You know, you are a human being and the patient is important, yes, but the disease, the patient and the family come together, they are all part of the same thing. And the group I talked with said they had forgotten that, they had honestly forgotten it and had never really thought about that. They were so busy with books, pens, computers you know.

Another felt that by informing future professionals they were helping the next generation of carers

> It's too late for us but we may be helping the next one.

The idea of having focused and protected time in which they talk about their own needs was again raised. One carer put it this way:

> I managed to shall we say, by me talking I got something off my chest, where before at home, you know, perhaps someone would come in—very seldom a doctor puts in an appearance—but you know no one really wants to listen to you. No one else was interested but this group of young people were very interested and, you know, it was the fact that I could get it all out. That's the main thing, get it all out in the open.

The opportunity to 'unload' angry feelings was identified by another carer as being of real value in the meeting with the students:

> I found it very helpful, therapeutic, because I hadn't realised that I was holding within me a lot of anger about medical care and the hospital . . . and so it was the first time I had an opportunity for medical people to listen and I unloaded quite a lot of my personal feelings about it.

Part of the reason for this was outlined by another carer as being due to having undisturbed and protected time, something that clearly was not a feature in the hospital:

> There were no interruptions, no bleepers going off or buzzers, nobody knocking on the door.

One of the concerns that we had had when deciding to involve carers in student education was their vulnerability. Our experience of working with families of people with terminal illness meant that, while not wanting to 'protect' the carers, we were uncertain about how students might handle sensitive issues. There was a real possibility that the carers might become distressed, which would be upsetting for them and the students. However we have found that, although carers do sometimes become tearful when recounting aspects of their loved one's illness or of their own bereavement, the students show a maturity in handling the situation. One carer expressed it as follows:

> I was upset, emotionally upset, and they coped with that very well and I didn't feel at all anxious about it. They didn't try and take it away from you which I think is very

important. They allowed you to be as you wanted to be and I thought that was a great strength.

Another carer said:

There was a lady [a student] sitting next to me and she quietly handed me a tissue and I apologised and they didn't look embarrassed.

Clearly then, our fears about 'exposing' carers or increasing their distress were not realized. Students were able to behave both sensitively and appropriately, and carers both enjoyed meeting the students and felt they could relate to them easily. This seems to be one way in which future professionals can be prepared for the 'messy world of practice' and have an opportunity to talk about the experience and knowledge gained to each other and to their course tutors.

An experience of involving carers in postgraduate inter-professional education

Our experience of involving carers in postgraduate inter-professional education was quite different. Here we will draw on our involvement in a postgraduate project involving inter-professional teams from four clinical settings—palliative care, elderly care, elderly mental health, and primary care—in Southampton (Report for NHSE South and West 1997). Unlike the undergraduate workshops described above, the carers' contribution was not central to the aims of this project. The focus of this project was a workshop intended to promote multi-professional, multi-agency learning. The workshop format involved the discussion of case studies within each clinical team. The plenary discussion offered the opportunity for the teams to learn from each other.

During the first phase of this postgraduate project, carers were invited to contribute their perspectives on care-giving in the plenary discussions. This was by its nature a very limited contribution. Because our work on the undergraduate workshops was developing at the same time, and the impact of the carers' contribution was so significant, a more central role for carers was built into the next phase of the postgraduate project.

This time, each team brought along a carer from the same clinical setting to the workshop. The intention was that the carer would form part of the team and participate equally in the discussions, which centred on the case studies. However, this proved to be unworkable. The clinical teams found it difficult to discuss issues openly in front of the carer. The carers also had different perceptions about their role within the group. Their experience of care-giving was very personal, whereas discussion around the case study needed to be much broader. Both the clinical team and the carer found this frustrating. One way around this problem was to enable the carers, working in a small group of their own, to consider their contributions to professional education. These views were fed back and discussed within the plenary session.

Creating a safe framework for learning from carers

Safety and sustainability are key issues to consider when engaging carers in supporting students' learning. We consider the reasons for this here and then in the final
section suggest guidelines for good practice, which address the issues.

There are several reasons why attention should be paid to the creation and maintenance of a safe framework for learning. First, effective learning can only take place
when the participants, in this case the students, carers, and facilitators, all feel suffi-
ciently safe. Risk-taking often enhances learning but must be taken within a framework that is explicit and secure. Students themselves worry about imposing on, or
upsetting, carers. Pill and Tapper-Jones (1993) describe the family case study programme in Cardiff, where students visit their assigned families at monthly intervals to
follow a newborn baby's development and discuss this with the baby's mother.
Although the vast majority of mothers found participation in this study to be an
enjoyable experience, students often expressed concerns about imposing on the
families. In our own experience, students seek reassurance that support is offered to
carers after the workshops, especially the carers who had been upset or emotional
during the story-telling. Indeed, as we observed earlier, students themselves may come
with personal or work experience of the issues raised by carers and may hear stories
that re-awaken earlier distress or resonate with current personal difficulties.

Second, because we have a duty of care to patients, carers, and students, it would be
unethical to embark on such an educational process without safeguards. Recalling difficult experiences is often painful for carers; sometimes the emotion expressed is anger
against the 'system' and/or the professionals. Students may find this distressing. They
may feel they have to defend their professional group. If this occurs and remains
unchallenged or not discussed, at best, learning will not be effective and, at worst,
confrontation and hostility can occur. The parent teachers involved in setting up the
Minnesota programme were very aware of this potential problem and (Blasco *et al.*
1999, p.697):

> ... made it clear that they in no way wanted the experience to be a 'doctor-bashing'
> session but rather a positive insightful experience, regardless of how positive or negative
> the family's past interactions may have been.

The carers too are embarking on an exercise that may lead them in a direction they
had not expected. In our undergraduate programme, because the interaction with
each new group is different, even those who have done it before may find themselves
focusing on a raw area this time. As their own situation changes over time, with
further deterioration in the person they are caring for, for example, or a changing
experience of bereavement, they may find their emotions nearer the surface. Current
carers acting as teachers are likely to have an ongoing relationship with the service
sector and it is important in their teaching experience to enhance rather than make
those relationships more difficult.

Third, carers come with very personal experiences. If students are to learn to extrap-
olate from unique situations to health and social care in general, they need to be able
to listen attentively and empathically to the carer, but to move away from the specifics

of that carer's situation and to translate that into lessons for their future role in caring as a professional.

Fourth, we have learnt from our own experience in the postgraduate project that clarity of the carers' role within the educational event is crucial. In our undergraduate workshops, carers are explicitly asked to tell their story. Questions surrounding teamwork relate to the specific experience that carer had undergone or was still experiencing. In the postgraduate project, carers were asked to participate as a member of the team in discussing a paper-case study This raised issues about the different perceptions of the carers and professionals about each others' roles in the team. Some of the carers who attended felt that they were there to 'teach' the professionals 'how to do it better', whilst others found it difficult to move away from their specific experience in order to participate in discussion of the hypothetical situation. Professionals felt constrained by the carers' presence. It is a moot point whether carers can be, or can perceive themselves to be, part of the 'team'. In this project, the lack of clarity about the carers' role within the educational event led to confusion.

Fifth, facilitators also need to have the balance between risk and safety maintained for themselves if they are to promote learning. Our experience has been with engaging carers in inter-professional sessions where there is the added dimension of teachers from the different health and social work professions collaborating in an educational event. But even where it is a uniprofessional session, with one facilitator, the same applies. The teacher must feel confident that s/he can use the unexpected as material for learning and that there are ways of supporting a distressed carer or student.

Sustainability is important because if engaging carers in teaching is marking a cognitive shift in health and social care education, it cannot be undertaken as a one-off exercise. Securing an appropriate environment, whether the learning takes place in an institution or in the carers' homes, recruitment and support of carers requires planning and an infrastructure. Our experience shows the value of carers, particularly in inter-professional education, since their concerns seldom involve just one profession's activities, and problems often occur because of the lack of collaboration between services. However this may add a further layer to the logistics—that of co-ordinating different programmes for the different professional qualifying courses.

Guidelines for good practice

1 Commit to developing an infrastructure that can sustain and support the initiative. On the institutional side, the Minnesota project has a programme director organizing and co-ordinating the experience in a way that integrates it with other clinical and teaching elements of their course (Blasco *et al.* 1999). In our own programme we have drawn on the fact that the medical members of the teaching team have clinical responsibilities in the hospice, and the nursing and social work members of the teaching team were in the past in practice there. Fortunately this gives confidence to those in the service, who are usually recruiting carers for us, that the teachers can be relied upon to generate a safe enough environment, and provides an easy channel

for feedback on any issues that carers subsequently raise about their participation that they have not voiced at the time.

Where carers are engaged in longer-term caring than is usually the case in palliative care, carer organisations themselves may organise recruitment and support in partnership with the educational sector. CRAC provides an example of an organisation which is both seeking and responding to opportunities (Soliman and Butterworth 1998).

2 Clear and thorough briefing is essential. This is equally important for learners and the carers. The learners need clarity about the purpose of the contact with, or input of, the carers, and it may be helpful, as in our undergraduate programme, to frame this around particular questions to give a focus. Carers also need clarity about why they have been asked to contribute and what it is the students need to learn from their experience of care-giving. However it is really important that carers tell their stories as they are, to reflect the messy world of practice. Any attempt to train the carers undervalues their local knowledge and diminishes the richness of that experience.

3 It is important to ensure that the interaction between students and carers take place in a safe setting. If the students are meeting carers in their own homes, or in a situation where the facilitator is not part of the group, it is important to recognize openly the students' possible apprehensions and consider strategies for meeting any difficulties. It is also important for facilitators to communicate their confidence in the ability of the learners to handle an encounter that, because of its nature, cannot be planned to the last detail. However learners need the confidence, whether in the lecture room or distant from it, that the facilitators can 'hold' the situation, or help the students 'hold' it, and will engage them without over-exposing them.

4 The students need to know that the facilitators will make the environment safe for the carers also. This is where welcoming the carers, making the environment as non-threatening as possible, ensuring that they are clear about why they are there, providing support during the session if needed, and setting time boundaries, all contribute to a safe framework for engaging carers in education.

5 After a powerful encounter, as these often are, debriefing is essential. For the students it is important to set the carers' input into a broader framework and to have the opportunity to reflect on any resonance in their personal experience. For carers, this may be done at a formal session afterwards (Blasco *et al.* 1999) or informally over a cup of coffee, as in our project.

6 Those who develop these learning experiences are often enthusiasts. In order to sustain these initiatives, and to maintain a sense of freshness for themselves, it is important to have opportunities to reflect with all those involved with the initiatives on how it is progressing. This often requires good links with the clinical team and others who may be involved in the care-giving process.

7 Evaluation by students and carers must form a basis for continuing reflection on the value and place of this experience in the curriculum. Ultimately there must be an evaluation of the impact of such sessions on patient care and family care.

Conclusion

In real life, carers are untrained and unselected. The inherent honesty in allowing carers to share their stories as they wish allows the students to experience practice as it is in reality. It also helps to shatter the illusion that patients' lives can be 'tidied up' or 'sanitized' in any way. This means that identical 'lessons' cannot be reproduced at each contact, whether in an institutional setting or in the carer's home, but it is the authenticity of the carers' experience that had a profound impact on the students. Here the facilitators play a key role in helping students to reflect on those experiences and learn from them, and in promoting the cognitive shift that will enable students to continue to value carers' local knowledge equally, alongside the professional knowledge they will develop in education and practice. Involving carers in professional education requires careful planning and facilitation—and a commitment to partnership with those who use services. In our experience this partnership appears to benefit all concerned, not only carers and students but also those running the workshops.

Acknowledgement

The authors would like to acknowledge the work of Richard Hillier and Colin Coles in developing and sustaining the undergraduate interprofessional workshops described in this chapter.

References

Barry, B. and Henderson, A. (1996). Nature of decision-making in the terminally ill patient. *Cancer Nursing* **19**, (5), 384–391.

Blasco, P. A., Kohen, H., and Shapland, C. (1999). Parents-as-teachers: design and establishment of a training programme for paediatric residents. *Medical Education* **33**, 695–701.

Coles, C. (1996). Undergraduate education and palliative care. *Palliative Medicine* **10**, 93–98.

Coles, C., Mountford, B., Hillier, R., Sheldon, F., Turner, P., and Wee, B. Undergraduate professional education: the evaluation of a model. (In preparation.)

Department of Health (1999). *Caring for carers: a national strategy for carers.* Department of Health, London

ENB (1996) *Learning from each other.* English National Board for Nursing, Midwifery and Health Visiting. London.

Eraut, M. (1994). *Developing professional knowledge and competence.* The Falmer Press, London.

Field, D., Douglas, C., Jagger, C., and Dand, P. (1995). Terminal illness: views of patients and their lay carers. *Palliative Medicine* **9**, 45–54.

Gibbs, G. (1992) *Improving the quality of student learning.* Technical and Educational Services Ltd., Bristol.

Hajioff, D. and Birchall, M. (1999). Medical students in ENT outpatient clinics: appointment time, patient satisfaction and student satisfaction. *Medical Education,* **33**, 669–673.

Harvath, T. A., Archbold, P. G., Stewart, B. J., Godow, S., Kirschling, J. M., and Miller, L. L. (1994). Establishing a partnership with family carers. *Journal of Gerontological Nursing,* **20**, 29–35.

Hendry, G. D., Schrieber, L., and Bryce, D. (1999). Patients teach students: partners in arthritis education. *Medical Education*, 33, 674–677.

Higginson, I., Wade, A., and McCarthy, M. (1990). Palliative care: views of patients and their families. *British Medical Journal*, 301, 277–81.

National Council for Hospice and Specialist Palliative Care Services (1985). *Specialist palliative care: a statement of definitions.* Occasional Paper 8, October 1995, London.

NHSE South and West (1997). *Report for Working together and learning together*

Nolan, M., Grant, G., and Keady, J. (1996). *Understanding family care.* Open University Press, Buckingham.

Pill, R. M. and Tapper-Jones, L. M. (1993). An unwelcome visitor? The opinions of mothers involved in a community-based undergraduate teaching project. *Medical Education* 27, 238–244.

Schön, D. (1987). *Educating the reflective practitioner.* Jossey-Bass, San Francisco.

Schultz, C. L., Smyrnios, K. X., Gribich, C. F., and Schultz, N. C. (1993). Caring for family caregivers in Australia: a model of professional support. *Ageing and Society*, 13, 1–25.

Soliman, A. and Butterworth, M. (1998). Why carers need to educate professionals. *Journal of Dementia Care.* May/June, 26–27.

Stacy, R. and Spencer, J. (1999). Patients as teachers: a qualitative study of patients' views on their role in a community-based undergraduate project. *Medical Education*, 33, 688–694.

Tope, R. (1998). *Meeting the challenge: introducing service users and carers into the education equation.* CAIPE Bulletin No. 15. UK Centre for the Advancement of Interprofessional Education.

Turner, P., Sheldon, F., Coles, C., Hillier, R., Mountford, B., Radway, P. *et al.* (2000) Listening to and learning from the family carer's story. *Journal of Interprofessional Care*, 14, 387–395.

Twigg, J. and Atkin, K. (1994). *Carers' perceived: policy and practice in informal care.* Buckingham, Open University Press.

Vanclay, L. (ed.) (1996). *Involving users in professional education.* CAIPE Bulletin No.12. UK Centre for the Advancement of Interprofessional Education.

Wykurz, G. (1999). Patients in medical education: from passive participants to active partners (commentary). *Medical Education*, 33, 634–636.

Chapter 9

The future: interventions and conceptual issues

Caroline Ellis-Hill and Sheila Payne

In order to look into the future it is necessary to look back and learn from others. During this century, European, North American, and some Asian countries such as Japan, will face serious challenges by their ageing populations, particularly as projections indicate rapid rises in those surviving to live over 85 years in the early decades of this century. As many older people live longer with chronic illnesses, the challenges will be: who will provide supportive care? While the responses of different countries vary in the nature and funding of health and social care systems, they are all based on the assumption that the majority of care will be provided by family members. This raises the important point that for increasing numbers of older people there will be nobody who can provide informal care, perhaps due to changing family patterns such as childlessness, marital breakdown, or geographical mobility. However, these issues are largely beyond the remit of this book. The experience of informal carers has been the topic of this book. In this final chapter we aim to draw together and highlight common themes that have been running through this book. These will form key conceptual issues and will be discussed in-depth. These concepts will then be used to suggest potential future interventions that could be provided by health and social care professionals.

Throughout this book the authors have recognized that the definitions of care and related concepts are influenced by, and influence, social and academic changes. All of the contributors have a clinical background and the theories they have developed are deeply rooted in practice. They have provided a broad background knowledge of the area, as well as highlighting current issues in research. The studies have drawn on a wide range of methodological approaches and varied in the methods used. They range from analysis at the macro level, with Lee's national survey with over 13 000 respondents, to the micro level, such as Ellis-Hill's in-depth analysis of the experiences of 10 spouses following their partners' stroke. It is interesting to note that although many differing approaches have been used, similar themes can been drawn from the evidence presented throughout the book. A key aspect of all of the studies has been the interest in exploring the psychological and social issues related to caring, and this chapter will continue to focus on those areas. Questions remain about the direction of future research—consumer involvement in research is now seen to be desirable.

Therefore, future research needs to draw on more participatory models, such as action research in which carers are able to collaborate in setting the research agenda, designing the project, and assisting with analysis.

The term carer came into common usage in the 1970s (Heaton 1999) and ideas about its role were developed largely from a professional perspective. In England and Wales a sizeable proportion of the 580 000 deaths each year have an identifiable terminal period. With the emergence of more people living with a chronic illness at home, and the trend to facilitate dying at home, the term 'carer' was developed to include family and friends—informal or primary carers. Family and friends are now seen to be the primary providers of care, with health and social care professionals supporting this informal network. The development of the term informal carer from a professional perspective has influenced the definition of caring. As it was based on the work of health carers, it is often defined in terms of the work or physical activity carried out by the informal carer. For example legislation to support carers such as the *Carers (Recognition and Services) Act 1995* (Department of Health and Social Services Inspectorate 1996) has defined carers as those providing 'regular and substantial care'. It has also affected the perception of caring in that, because professionals equate it with their own jobs, they recognize that it must be very stressful and burdensome to be working 24 h a day. There has been a great deal of literature on the burden of care and over time it appears to have become one of the key theoretical concepts related to caring.

Although recognizing that there are burdensome aspects to caring, the authors in this book have highlighted that this is a limited way to view the caring situation. In many studies, participants have reported that the physical aspects of caring are often the easiest ones to cope with and manage. Ensuring that there is availability of appropriate services and adequate resources is only the first step in helping to support carers provide care at home. Services need to be introduced at a pace and at a time that is acceptable and comfortable for patients and carers, and not when crises loom. The timing of initiating these support services is very complex within palliative care, as predicting the speed of decline in physical ability is difficult. Patients and carers may be very reluctant to anticipate deterioration, as it reminds them that the end of life may be near. There needs to be a greater understanding of how patients and carers experience dilemmas in seeking or accepting help.

It is often the emotional and personal changes in their lives that are the ones that cause them most distress. Also Nolan (Chapter 2) highlights that there are many positive aspects of caring, which cannot be explained by the 'burden' model. Twigg and Aitkin (1994) caution against viewing caring in terms of an extension of the professional role as this can lead to a medical or pathological model of family caring. This could lead to health and social care professionals carrying out interventions that are purely practically based rather than also addressing emotional aspects that affect the caring situation. Also, the close identification with the formal nursing role may place limitations on carers themselves, in that they may use their experience of nursing as their template for action. Rose (Chapter 4), highlighted that carers often feel that they should be sympathetic and supportive of the cared-for at all times (as would be expected of nursing staff) and felt guilty and ashamed when they could no longer maintain this unrealistic expectation.

The authors in this book have presented many alternative concepts related to family caring. Three key features in their research have been the need to focus on the perspective of the person providing the care, the recognition that understanding has to be based on a consideration of the wider everyday life issues that impact on the caring situation, and the temporal nature of caring. These three aspects will be discussed in turn. First, the authors have recognized that a carer's perception of their role is inherent in understanding their behaviour and their emotional state. Smith (Chapter 5) noted that spouses caring for their partners with a terminal illness often do not see themselves as carers, but as husbands or wives. It is only when we take the perspective of the person themselves, that we realize the complexity of the situation, and the importance of personal and individual meaning. Each carer has a unique response to their situation due to their own individual past and present circumstances. Second, Rose (Chapter 4) noted that informal caring differs from formal caring in that it is not episodic, but it is the fabric of everyday life. Home is the setting for family caregiving. People with a chronic illness live in the community with their illness and in terminal illness, people spend 90% of their last year of life at home (Seale and Cartwright 1994). Therefore the focus within caring research should be the everyday life of the family rather than merely specific medical or nursing aspects. This approach also highlights the all-encompassing nature of being in a caring situation. Third, we need to recognize the temporal aspect of caring and the need to carry out longitudinal studies to see how the situation changes over time. People pass through many transitions: becoming a carer, being a carer, and no longer being a carer. These transitions may or may not link with physical caring as will be discussed below.

In order to address the psychological and social issues that cannot be explained by the burden model of caring, we feel that it is important to recognize that caring involves making, maintaining, and ending relationships. Nolan (Chapter 2) found that 80% of caregivers had a satisfying relationship, showing that caring was a meaningful activity not just a burden. He highlighted that emotional well-being of the carer was more closely related to the quality of relationships than the amount of time that was spent caring, and that caring situations with no positive feedback were probably the most difficult to manage. Cox and Dooley (1996) reported that carers who found their situation easier, cared for people who were seen to try as much a possible, provided emotional support to the caregiver, were appreciative, had a sense of humour, were fun to be with, and did not complain. Whereas those who found their situations more difficult cared for people who were seen to resist help, had no interest, were seen to be too demanding, or expected more than the caregiver could provide. Difficulty in a caregiving situation can be seen to relate as much to the types of relationships formed as the actual physical help provided.

The term carer is a relational concept. Carers only exist in relation to other people, be they the cared-for or the formal care workers they may be working alongside. We feel it is important to understand not only how relationships are maintained or changed through discourse and action at many different levels, but also how relationships influence individuals' thinking and future actions. We will discuss four key relationships: those between carers and the cared-for; carers and family and friends; carers and employers; and finally carers and the formal care professionals. These will be discussed in more detail below. Although we recognize the complexity of the social situations that impact on caregiving and how other relationships such as those between cared-for and professionals impact on the situation, our main focus will be the relationships formed by carers, as they are the focus of this book. Also, we recognize the inter-related aspects of the different relationships but have described them separately for ease of discussion.

Relationship with the cared-for

As Smith noted (Chapter 5), not all people considered by health professionals to be carers, actually define themselves as carers. The majority of respondents in Smith's study defined their position in terms of their relationship with the ill person rather than as a role or job. They saw their activity as being based on a desire to share with their partner, show love and concern, and repay them for care that had been given to them in the past. It was seen as a natural progression of the relationship they had built together, rather than an additional job that they had taken on. Rose (Chapter 4) also highlighted that relatives reported that they were caring because of love, duty, or previous promises, rather than because they felt they had to take on the job. It is interesting to note the differing social expectations of different generations described by Lee (Chapter 7). Within this national survey in Australia, the older age-group of women saw caring as a natural role for them and a repayment for past care; whereas the middle–aged women saw their caring role more in terms of a job—a valuable but unappreciated contribution to the countries health care system. Changes in the expectations that women will take up paid work may have a bearing on this.

By framing caring within relationships it is possible to consider how previous relationships may affect the situation. Rose (Chapter 4) noted the additional difficulty of caring for close family members in that previous relationships impact on the present situation. A daughter mentioned that it was difficult to give personal care to her father, who used always to be seen as a figure of authority. Another carer reported that she was having problems caring for her older sister, who had always wanted to be in control. Acknowledging previous relationships also highlights the additional pain of seeing a loved one becoming frustrated or suffering.

Many participants have commented on how their cared-for person has changed—and is no longer seen as the person the carer once knew. One of Rose's participants noted, 'It is heartbreaking, she was still my sister, but she wasn't' (Chapter 4). This has an impact on how carers see themselves in relation to the cared-for—they may take on a mothering role, where before they were a daughter, or a nursing role, where before they were a lover. This changes their own position and they may lose ways of defining themselves, which often they have had for many years. This can be very distressing. An extreme case can be seen in the effect of a relative being hospitalized following an acute injury and needing ventilation. As one of Sque's respondents (Chapter 6) said, 'When they go into places like this they don't feel as if they are yours anymore—you're outside looking in, as if they are nothing to do with you'. It can be seen that often within caring situations former relationships with the cared-for are compromised and challenged.

All of the authors noted the importance to carers of trying to maintain or rebuild this relationship. Maintaining the identity of the cared-for was important for carers. Carers spent a great deal of effort in social situations in helping the cared-for person maintain or regain their social standing by highlighting the preferences or choices they had made. Sque (Chapter 6) noted that decisions made by carers were often based on how the deceased would have wanted to have things managed or carried out. Being physically close to the cared-for appears to be important in maintaining the relationship. The majority of the participants felt the need to visit the cared-for if they were in hospital or in a home on a regular (usually daily) basis. Sque (Chapter 6) noted that the emotional and physical presence of being with, and seeing, the patient was often helpful to families. Carers practice a sense of vigilance and looked out for their loved-one. It appears that part of visiting the hospital was to find out what was happening and to ensure their relative had the best possible care. It was important to families to feel that the health professionals cared about their relative and valued them as a person. This was demonstrated by professionals' words, actions, and presence. For example, one of Sque's (Chapter 6) respondents felt that the nurses 'messing about' in the office were disrespectful, and another reported that he was distressed as he felt that his wife was treated as an abstract entity which the staff were performing on.

This aspect of caring and the need to maintain a relationship appeared to reach beyond physical caring in a temporal sense. As mentioned above, although people do not physically care while their loved-one is in hospital or in a home, they still have the need to maintain a caring relationship. Nolan (Chapter 2) noted the potential guilt expressed by relatives when their loved-one moves into a home. Sque (Chapter 6) noted the difficulty that carers faced in feeling the need to maintain a relationship with what was rationally perceived to be a ventilated corpse. Rose (Chapter 4) also noted the importance to carers, following the death of their loved-one, that they had discussed the future and could carry on in the future in a way that their loved one would have approved. It appears that caring relationships go on beyond death. Sque noted the distress experienced by a family who had been sent away from the hospital with a plastic bag of their loved-ones belongings wondering, 'What do we now?'. There was no recognition of an ongoing relationship with the loved-one and the need to maintain the identity of the person that had been lost. Sque also noted that, following the experience of intensive care and organ donation, families also appreciated the ability to say goodbye to nursing and hospital staff, and recognize the new relationships they had formed.

It appears that the perceptions of becoming a carer develop over time. Most of the participants in Smith's (Chapter 5) study were caring for less than a year. Those that readily identified with the term carer had often been caring for over a year. Those that defined themselves as a carer often had some pattern of caring throughout their lives, were therefore experienced, saw it as a valued role, and gained a great deal of satisfaction. They often found it difficult to talk about themselves and tended to talk in terms of 'us' or 'we' rather than 'I' or 'me'. Although this close identification with the cared-for was satisfying when the situation was stable, an exploration of relationships highlights that this may create difficulties when physical caring changes or ends. If the cared-for person moves into a residential home, is admitted to hospital, or dies, this close identification may create additional confusion as the carer tries to create a new identity as a non-carer. Sque noted that for one of her respondents, her sense of being a carer had become the complete part of identity following her mother's death she said, 'I've been leading someone else's life, my mothers I suppose' (Chapter 6). This situation was also highlighted by one of Lee's respondents who described how as a woman she had spent all her life looking after others and had one day 'woken up completely exhausted, [and found that] everything's gone—and you wonder who the hell are you? And where am I supposed to go from here?' (Chapter 7) There are many changes in the intimate relationships between cared-for and carer that have an emotional impact on caregiver and how they perceive themselves, and how they manage all the transitions of becoming, maintaining, and ending caring relationships. In the next section we will move on beyond the dyadic relationship to consider wider social factors that affect the caregiving situation.

Relationship with family and friends

Rose (Chapter 4) highlighted that there appears to be two main scenarios. Friends and relatives are either very supportive and good relationships are strengthened, or the carer is increasingly left to manage alone and becomes increasingly isolated. She noted that when friends were involved, they saw part of their role as to support the caregiver practically and emotionally but not necessarily to be closely involved in day-to-day caring. Family can become an important part of the caregiving situation, as one of Lee's respondents said, 'You can have the best medical help available but without the love and support from a loving family and friends you will not survive' (Chapter 7). It seems that the perceived support experienced by carer, rather than the number of friends or relatives available, has an effect on the emotional state of the carer. Rose noted that secondary carers were often aware of their different position, in that they could go back to their own homes and leave the caregiving situation. They did not appear to be so emotionally bound and talked more openly about the conflict between their own needs and the needs of the person they were caring for. The family may be the source of additional work for the carer as well as a source of support. Carers may have dependent children or other relatives that need their support. They may still have any domestic duties relating to other family members. Although this may impact on their main caring role, several carers noted that it was quite therapeutic to be able to maintain the normal routine of housework in the potentially stressful situation in which they found themselves (Rose Chapter 4 and Sque Chapter 6).

Family and friends are not only a source of direct support, but along with other social groups may provide the support and stimulus to undertake leisure, hobbies, and other social activities. Lee (Chapter 7) noted that time out and leisure was important in helping caregivers to cope. As one respondent noted, the time completely away had been a great rejuvenation to her health, both mental and physical. However, Lee noted that many older women felt unable to take short breaks away. They had a sense of regret that they had no time for themselves, and no opportunities for relaxation or enjoyment.

Relationship with employers and colleagues

Many participants of working age noted that the relationship that they had with their employers and work colleagues was a crucial factor in the caregiving situation. If employers were sympathetic and allowed flexible working, then a great weight was lifted from carers (Smith Chapter 5). Several carers noted that going to work was important to them, in that they felt that it gave them a break. They saw it as time for themselves when they could make the most of the companionship of their colleagues.

However, if employers were not sympathetic, then this added to carers' emotional distress. Rose (Chapter 4) described the strain experienced by those who were trying to balance the caring and working role, and felt that they were doing neither to their own satisfaction. Some respondents were also distressed as they felt that they were letting down work colleagues. Some carers were also affected by the social expectation that time off from work could only be given for personal health reasons. Rose described a case where a wife had to be labelled as suffering from anxiety, so that her GP could write a sick note. As Rose noted, this false record could affect her employment prospects in the future.

If carers felt they could no longer continue to work, they not only faced the potential loss of companionship, familiarity, and sense of contributing to society, they also had to face the long-term financial and employment implications (Lee Chapter 7). If they were not financially secure they had to rely on benefits, leading to an additionally restricted life style. Lee noted that a break away from work could affect the persons future careers prospects.

By considering the caregiving situation in terms of relationships, it can be seen that carers may be facing a myriad of changes in relationships at many differing levels, which have long-term implications for themselves and their lives. Each person will have a different set of past and present circumstances that they have to face. In the previous sections we have aimed to highlight the potential complexity of the situation that carers are facing. It is not that we feel that it is the role of health professionals to address all of these issues but to recognize that an appreciation of the wider individual circumstances of the person they are working alongside. This may help them to develop interventions that are more practicable and helpful in the daily life of carers. We will now turn our attention to the impact that relationships with health and social care professionals have on the caregiving situation.

Relationships with health and social care professionals

Health care professionals work within a culture where two key factors influence their relationships with carers. The first factor is that the legitimate focus for the professional is seen to be the cared-for person rather than the carer. The second factor is the fact that professionals often hold the power within these relationships, as they control access to technical and financial resources and control understanding of the systems involved. We will discuss each of these in more details

As mentioned previously it is widely accepted that carers will put the cared-for person's needs before their own. Within a health care setting professionals work closely with the ill person and involve carers as they feel necessary. This may vary between chronic illness and terminal care settings. Since the inception of the hospice movement, there is more of an emphasis on support for the families of terminally ill people (Seale 1989), whereas in services provided for those living with a chronic illness, carers are rarely the focus for concern. The position of carers is highlighted by Smith (Chapter 5) when she notes that the family caregivers' stories are often embedded in patients' stories and they do not expect to talk about themselves or their own feelings. She also notes that this feeling may be more acute in those caring for a partner with a terminal illness. Smith highlights that the caregiver's own story was often hidden. Her respondents reported that if they did speak with health professionals it was usually to discuss the welfare and care of the patients. The only personal access they had was to have a few words at the beginning or end of a visit, and these tended to be general, polite questions related to how they were coping or managing overall. Sheldon *et al.* (Chapter 8) note that in the education of health professionals, patients have always received far more focus from professional students than their carers, although they acknowledge that there is more emphasis on family and society in social work education.

It has been highlighted that when individuals first find themselves in a caring situation they are often unsure of the practical aspects of caring and they turn to health professionals for advice and guidance. As noted by Sque (Chapter 6), when relatives were admitted to hospital, carers lost control to professionals as they were functioning outside their familiar world. Over time, as Smith (Chapter 5) noted, they may become the link between health professionals and the cared-for by being present in medical and nursing consultations. However, from the case studies described by Sheldon *et al.* (Chapter 8) it is apparent that caregivers, even when working alongside health professionals, may not know about medical terminology, disease process, treatment, side-effects, and prognosis. Also they are often unaware of the different systems of health and social care, and differing policy and funding arrangements. We are not suggesting that caregivers need to necessarily have all of this knowledge, but there appears be a power imbalance in that professionals retain a knowledge base to which carers do not appear to have access. Again there may be differences in services provided for people with terminal and chronic illnesses. Smith (Chapter 5) found that her respondents reported that they knew who to contact and had established to their own satisfaction who they should contact in different circumstances. This is often not the case within the services provided for those with a chronic illness (Ellis-Hill Chapter 3).

Carers do gain more knowledge over time. They become knowledgeable about the practical needs of their cared-for person and daily procedures that work best within the home. This has been defined as local knowledge, as opposed to the cosmopolitan (general and technical) knowledge held by professionals (Harvath *et al.* 1994). They may also become extremely proficient and knowledgeable about technical aspects of care. Sheldon *et al.* (Chapter 8) note that several carers reported that they became annoyed when professional carers 'took over' and their expertise was not recognized or accepted. Professional knowledge is often privileged over local knowledge when decisions are taken about care. This was highlighted by the respondents described by

Rose (Chapter 4) who felt that they did not have control over the situation and had to fight to get things done for their relative. This power imbalance was also noted by Sheldon *et al.* (Chapter 8) when describing professional education. They described how the students felt that they had not had the chance to meet family members before the training sessions. This was despite having already met patients with relatives on hospital wards. Sheldon *et al.* concluded that they apparently did not have the insight or encouragement to recognize that relatives are important people to talk to. It appears that within the present health culture carers are hidden from and excluded from the processes of formal care.

Why is there a disparity between what health and social care professionals would like to provide and the experience of carers? We feel that one of Sheldon *et al.*'s carer respondents highlighted the issue in this piercing quote:

> They need to be given experience of human feelings. When you train you become a robot—they [healthcare staff] put you down this lane as if you do this, you do that, you do the other. You've got to do this by a certain date and they forget that you aren't just a number. You know, you are a human being and the patient is important, yes, but the disease, the patient and the family come together, they are all part of the same thing. And the group I talked with said they had forgotten that, they had honestly forgotten it and had never really thought about that. They were so busy with books, pens, computers you know.

Implications for practice

So what are the implications of care when considering relationships within the caring situation? There are several interlinking aspects, but the primary aspect appears to be the need to recognize and redress the power differential between health care provider and family carer. We recognize that this is a very difficult aspect to achieve and necessitates individual, organizational, and social change, but we hope to highlight a few key aspects that could be addressed.

Recognize power differential between health care provider and family carer

As Sheldon *et al.* note (Chapter 8), professional practice—especially in the care of families living with chronic and terminal illnesses—is messy and confusing, with many problems that defy technical solutions. Practitioners, as well as carers, have to deal with a complex and challenging world. This has been highlighted in the previous paragraphs. Sheldon *et al.* noted that when working on the wards and listening to family carers, staff have pre-set agendas into which requests, queries, and the concerns of carers are assimilated. As one nurse, reflecting on a time when she was listening to a carer, said, 'I was assessing, starting to work out what sort of things I was going to provide because that is my role' (Chapter 8). Health care professionals are trained and supported to 'do' for others, to take action, to respond. Often the plans we make are based on our own previous knowledge and experience. Sheldon *et al.* suggest that we need a cognitive shift to be able to recognize that plans should be based on carers' experiences and local knowledge, as well as our own knowledge. As they note, it may be very difficult at first to accept this change (and reduction) in power and, second, to be able to sustain the change while still maintaining a professional contribution.

They suggest that the first step in valuing another's contribution is to be able to listen and follow the carer's agenda, rather than feeling the need to ask routine medical and nursing questions. They suggest that it is also important to confirm and clarify aspects with carers rather than jumping to conclusions As one student mentioned, she aims not to be so clinical but to find out their (patients') needs and talk to them more. Also, professionals need to be able to feel happy with listening to aspects, which at first may not seem to be 'relevant'. As noted above, if the professionals want to support carers, they need to be able to assess all the differing facets of the caregiving situation that the carer feels is important to them.

As Smith (Chapter 5) noted, carers do not expect professionals to ask them about their own concerns. Professionals need to create an organizational structure where carers are given time to discuss their own needs and concerns, before action is taken by professionals that affects the caregiving situation. Smith noted that, although carers may know who to contact, they are quite reticent about approaching professionals and often wait until the professionals contact them. This suggests that professionals should systematically initiate meetings between themselves and carers to encourage carers to become involved.

Developing a working relationship

Having heard and recognized the differences in the perceptions of the world of the professional and family, Smith (Chapter 5) highlights that it is important to acknowledge that carers have rights and needs, and that they are explicitly defined within the care plan. This partnership model has been highlighted in the Carers National Strategy (DOH 1999)

Developing a working relationship not only enables the health professional to develop an intervention that is more suited to the caregiving situation, but also helps to support the caregiver in the stressful situation they find themselves in. As mentioned previously, they may be in a state of flux and many relationships are changing. By listening, the professional validates the experience of the caregiver (Langer 1993), building their confidence. If health professionals see an important aspect of their work as building and maintaining good working relationships, it can be seen that it is important that, if the plans are agreed with carers, that they happen, because, as Rose highlights (Chapter 4), if they do not, this is not only inconvenient for the carer but damages the relationship between professional and carer.

In order for care to be collaborative it is in important that carers are kept informed of anything that affects their relative, as this will impact on the caregiving situation. Sque (Chapter 6) noted that the amount of knowledge family members felt they had received about the care given to relatives had long-term effects on bereavement. Also, it is helpful to recognize that carers are constantly monitoring the cared-for's situation, and recognition of the value of this work will support a good working relationship.

Long-term nature of the working relationship

We have noted the long-term nature of chronic and terminal illness, and the tempo-ral aspect of caring. It is therefore important to recognize the need for long-term rela-tionships between health and social care professionals and carers, so that appropriate responses to changes in the caregiving situation can be made. We would suggest that a high quality service would be one that enables the carer to form a relationship with the same professional or small group of professionals over this length of time. This gives a chance for good working relationships to develop, making it more likely that carers will seek support when it is needed. Smith (Chapter 5) noted that carers get information from those with whom they have most contact and have formed the closest relationships with, rather then approaching a particular health professional appropriate for their specific need.

Support through transitions in caring

We have also noted that it is important to recognize that caring relationships extend beyond physical caring relationships, and that carers may be at different points in their caring relationships: they need differing types of intervention depending on whether they are taking up, maintaining, or ending relationships. Professionals need to assess a carer's level of expertise, rather than making assumptions. Nolan (Chapter 2) also suggests that professionals need to support carers in making choices about whether to take up caring, continue caring, or give up caring. In the present social and political climate it may be extremely difficult to provide such a choice. We also recog-nize that a caring relationship is maintained after physical caring has ended. Sheldon *et al.* (Chapter 8) highlight the importance of continuing to visit even if there seems little in the way of treatment which can be given

Maintaining the identity of the cared-for

Also as noted in a previous section, maintaining the identity of the cared-for is impor-tant for relationships between caregiver and cared-for. Family carers find it very sup-portive if their loved ones are treated with dignity, propriety, and care. Again this goes beyond death, as Sque (Chapter 6) noted that it was important to family members that they knew that organ retrieval was carried out with care and gentleness.

Wider range of interventions

Nolan (Chapter 2) suggested that not only do we need a reconfiguration of the rela-tionship between professionals and family carers, we need a reconceptualization of the aims and objectives of interventions designed to support family carers. He suggested that we should move toward more innovative programmes of support for family carers that promote satisfactions in caregiving. Ellis-Hill suggested that we should analyse caring situations further and focus on both carer and cared-for, so that the quality and meaning of life for both is enhanced.

Future interventions include asking carers to work with students. Sheldon *et al.* (Chapter 8) note the power of the message provided by carers themselves when they note that the authenticity that carers themselves leads to attitude change which cannot be communicated by the facilitators alone.

Conclusion

We have highlighted several ways forward in health and social care practice, but we do not suggest that these are *the* only answers. We hope this chapter has highlighted the complexity and competing factors that influence the caring situation. We hope we have introduced new ideas, which will help each practitioner, manager, and researcher to reflect on their work and develop a suitable way forward. We would like to end the chapter by highlighting that individuals alone cannot change this situation, and that wider social influences have a bearing on future possibilities. We would like to present two examples. Lee (Chapter 7) noted that 70% of caregivers in Australia and the UK are women and it is often assumed that it is 'naturally' a women's role to care. Government agencies and employers see caregiving and its conflicts as a primarily private issue and a women's problem, which is not relevant to employment conditions or the provision of heath and welfare services (Gonyea and Googins 1992). These social barriers need to be recognized and acted upon if carers are to have a genuine choice in caring. Also, within the health service within the UK there is a desire to be able to demonstrate and measure practical concrete interventions, which can be seen to contribute to the evidence base for health care. The development of clinical pathways, aimed to provide comparative and equitable care based on diagnosis, is also another example of the desire to provide a systematic approach to health care. These developments, although understandable, challenge professionals in being able to provide truly individualised care based on the often unmeasurable aspects of a collaborative caring partnership.

References

Cox, E. O. and Dooley, A. C. (1996). Care-receivers' perception of their role in the care process. *Journal of Gerontological Social Work*, 26, (1/2), 133–52.

Department of Health and Social Services Inspectorate (1996). *Carers (Recognition and Services) Act 1995: practice guidance*. Department of Health/Social Services Inspectorate, London.

Department of Health (1999). *The carers national strategy*. The Stationery Office, London.

Gonyea, J. G. and Googins, B. K. (1992). Linking the worlds of work and family: beyond the productivity trap. *Human Resource Management*, 31, 209–226.

Harvath, T. A., Archbold, P. G., Stewart, B. J., Godow, S., Kirschling, J. M., Miller, L. L. *et al.* (1994). Establishing partnerships with family caregivers: local and cosmopolitan knowledge. *Journal of Gerontological Nursing*, 20, (2), 29–35.

Heaton, J. (1999). The gaze and visibility of the carer: a Foucauldian analysis of the discourse of informal care. *Sociology of Health and Illness*, 21, (6), 759–777.

Langer, S. R. (1993). Ways of managing the experience of caregiving for elderly relatives. *Western Journal of Nursing Research*, 15, (5), 582–94.

Seale, C. and Cartwright, A. (1994). *The year before death*. Avebury, Aldershot.

Seale, C. (1989). What happens in hospices: a review of research evidence. *Social Science Medicine*, 28, (6), 551–559.

Twigg, J. and Atkin, K. (1994). *Carers perceived: policy and practice in informal care*. Open University Press, Buckingham.

Index